PHYSICAL THERAPY

and Rehabilitation *for*

ANIMALS

A GUIDE FOR THE CONSUMER

**Help Your Pet Overcome Disability, Maximize Recovery,
and Prevent Injury Through Knowledge and Guidance
from an experienced, trained animal health care professional**

SUSAN E. DAVIS, PT

joycare
onsite™

Handwritten inscription: To: Janet Bob — great friends & neighbors + in Memory of Jesse & Freddie ♡ All the best, Davispt (Sue)

PHYSICAL THERAPY AND REHABILITATION FOR ANIMALS:
A GUIDE FOR THE CONSUMER
Copyright © 2013 by Susan E. Davis, PT

Published by Joycare Media
Red Bank, NJ 07701

ISBN: 978-0-9892750-0-2

Cover and Interior Design by GKS Creative
Illustrations by K J Hempstead
Back cover photography by Tanya Breen

First Printing
Printed in the United States of America

Library of Congress Cataloging-in-Publication

Davis, Susan E., 1955-
        Physical therapy and rehabilitation for animals : a
        guide for the consumer / Susan E. Davis.
        p. cm.
        Includes index.
        "Help your pet overcome disability, maximize recovery
        and prevent injury through knowledge and guidance from
        an experienced, trained animal health care professional."
        ISBN 978-0-9892750-0-2
        ISBN 978-0-9892750-1-9

        1. Veterinary physical therapy.   I. Title.

SF925.D38 2013   636.089
                         QBI13-600074

"It is just like man's vanity and impertinence to call an animal dumb because it is dumb to his dull perceptions."
—MARK TWAIN

This book is dedicated to all of my past, present, and future animal patients and their devoted families.
And is in memory of "Pipsqueak."

TABLE of CONTENTS

- Ultrasound
- Heat versus Cold
- Extracorporeal Shock-Wave Therapy

- Range of Motion
- Stretching
- Joint Mobilization and Manipulation
- Traction
- Strengthening
- Functional Exercises
- Swimming

- Underwater Treadmills
- Land Treadmills
- Rails and Poles
- Physio-Rolls and Balls
- Balance and Rocker Boards

- Compensation and Symmetry
- Hip Dysplasia
- Cranial Cruciate Ligament Tears
- Patellar Luxation
- Hock Injuries
- Rotator Cuff
- Elbow Fractures
- Elbow Dysplasia

- Earth and Working Activities
- Walking as Therapy
- Injury Prevention
- Core Strengthening
- The Tables Are Turned!

ACKNOWLEDGMENTS

So many people and animals have given me opportunities and encouragement along the way. I recognize and thank the following:

John Bergmann, director of the Associated Humane Societies Popcorn Park Zoo, Forked River, NJ. Thank you for your support and your kindness and compassion for all of the animals.

Dr. Laney Baris, VMD, Popcorn Park Animal Clinic. The brightest, finest veterinarian I have seen, who appreciates the field of physical therapy and is open to utilizing its benefits to any and all species.

Dr. Steve Cudia, VMD, Veterinary Surgical Services. One of the first doctors to trust me with his post-surgery patients, and one who is always willing to take the time to communicate and share information.

Dr. Patrick Mahaney, VMD, integrative veterinarian and founder of California Pet Acupuncture and Wellness (CPAW), Inc. We met via Twitter and became fast friends and professional partners due to our shared passion for animals and physical rehabilitation.

Jana Rade, founder of the amazing blog *Dawg Business: It's Your Dog's Health*. Thank you for giving me the opportunity to write articles, thereby infecting me with the bug.

Carol Bryant, founder of FidoseofReality.com, dog lover of the highest order, fabulous writer of all things pet, and whose heart beats dog!

Donna Cardillo, nurse guru, speaker, and author, who has been a mentor to me over the years.

Bethany Brown, principal at The Cadence Group, and Amy Collins of New Shelves Distribution, for their expertise and for encouraging me to keep writing.

Angelina Ruggiero, canine swim expert, friend, and extraordinary dog momma.

Kathy Hogelin-Harrison, for allowing me to be photographed with her beautiful Weimaraners.

Beverly Tiemann, my mom, for her enduring love and wisdom.

Susan Tobier Rogove, my best pal, for her unending encouragement and valued advice.

Mark Davis, my beloved husband, for his love and patience.

Penelope, our darling Dachshund, for sharing me when I go to work to "help the sick doggies, kitties, bunnies ...."

FOREWORD

I met Limpy at a dog park. A young Lab, full of life. Even though it wasn't slowing him down much, he was clearly favoring his left hind leg. I asked what happened.

"He's torn a knee ligament," the owner said.

Having a dog with tattered ligaments in both knees myself, I inquired how they were going to treat Limpy.

"He already had a surgery," was the response. "He had a TPLO about year ago, but is still favoring the leg a bit."

Here's the thing. If Limpy had surgery a year ago, he was done recovering. What you saw is what you got—a lame dog. Could it be the doctors botched the surgery? That's one possibility. More likely though, Limpy didn't get the post-op physical therapy he needed.

Diet, exercise, physical therapy—these are unpopular options. They require effort. We don't want to work for things. Instead, we want a magic pill, or a magic surgery, that will fix everything quickly and easily. Unfortunately, things don't work that way.

When our dog, Jasmine, was going in for knee surgery, her vet stressed emphatically that what we do during recovery would make or break the success of the whole venture. We received detailed post-op instructions and were told to adhere to them religiously. Cold and warm compresses, passive range of motion (PROM) exercises, massage, and functional and strength exercises—all are critical to a successful outcome.

We did these things as if our lives depended on it. And yet, a disturbingly large number of owners bring their dogs in for knee surgery and don't receive any instructions for post-op care at all!

Physical therapy is not only crucial in the post-operative period, it can sometimes even replace surgery or drug therapy. Bodies are designed to move. In fact, that is the whole idea behind having a body, such as it is, in the first place. If you left your car sitting in the backyard, sooner or later you can expect the engine to seize up and the body to rust out. After some time of not going anywhere, the car is not going anywhere. Machines and bodies remain functional by performing the work they were designed for.

Moving properly is more important than you can imagine, not just for the injured area but for the body as a whole. As soon as something is not working properly, the rest of the body will do its best to compensate. That sounds like a good thing, until you think about the domino effect.

Once, my husband developed a wart on his foot. It was quite painful, so he did his best not to put any pressure on that spot. In no time at all, his leg was sore all the way up to the hip! It's no different when your dog has an injury or pain anywhere in its body. Problems like to snowball.

Keeping Jasmine healthy has been challenging, but I quickly realized that physical therapy was one of the best treatment options I could provide for her. Not only during post-op care, but also to deal with her injuries, keeping her arthritis in check, keeping her bodily systems working well, and even for her brain!

I met Susan Davis on my quest to learn all I could about what physical therapy could offer Jasmine, and which modalities or techniques would be best to use. You would be hard-pressed to find somebody who knows more about physical therapy than Susan. The best indicator of her expertise is how her animal patients respond to her, and how they improve under her care.

Some people have jobs, some have careers—for Susan, being a physical therapist is a calling.

When I found out she was going to write a book, I was thrilled that more people and pets were going to be able to benefit from her know-how. We need to know this stuff. Physical therapy can do a world of good not only when your dog is suffering from an orthopedic condition, but it can even help with rehabilitation of neurological and some medical conditions.

Jasmine is certainly grateful for all the things I've learned from Susan. Considering her medical history, there is a good chance Jasmine wouldn't have been with us today. But she is, and while the challenges never seem to end, she is full of life, enjoys her hikes, and wants to rumble with the healthiest of them.

What do I like the most about physical therapy? There is no downside. Performed properly, it can only do good.

Jana Rade
Dog health advocate and blogger
http://dawgbusiness.blogspot.ca

INTRODUCTION

Considering that freshman English composition was the subject that most threatened to derail my GPA and thus possibly deny admission to the physical therapy program I desperately wanted to attend, writing this or any book seemed improbable. I admit to taking an incomplete in the course and resuming it in the summer when I could guarantee my undivided attention to manage a decent grade. Yes, ultimately I was accepted to Northwestern University School of Physical Therapy in Chicago and have enjoyed a thirty-five-year career in this multifaceted field. Life is full of irony.

If I had been told in 1977 that I would eventually use my qualifications as a physical therapist to work with animals, it would have seemed ridiculous. There was little thought of physical therapy (PT) for animals, other than horses, until the late 1990s.

I've always loved animals, particularly dogs. In fact, I would admit to being passionate about them. When I became aware of a canine rehabilitation program at the University of Tennessee's Veterinary School, through Northeast Seminars, I was intrigued. By this point, I was in serious need of a new challenge and a chance to combine my professional skills and knowledge with a new patient population.

Having entered the PT field in the mid-1970s, more than fifty years after its origin, it was very exciting to begin study in the field of canine rehabilitation at its inception in the early 2000s. When I finally broke free of human patients at the end of 2007 and began a canine and small animal practice in early 2008, there was vast open territory to explore and develop.

From owning private physical therapy facilities and employing staff, I had a fresh desire to stay small and personal. Thus, the concept of providing animal PT on-site, in the pet's home, or another location, was born. At the same time, I did not want to be isolated but rather wanted to stay connected to other professionals. I also had a long-range goal to volunteer. Thus, I carved out one day per week from my new private practice to provide pro-bono physical therapy services to an animal shelter and zoo. Along with this great adventure came the opportunity to work "beyond canine" with multiple species in a unique role I never imagined possible.

New ground has been broken. I have stories to tell. I have information to share. This field is exploding and owners, guardians, and parents of animals need to understand the benefits of physical therapy to enable them to help their pets when the need arises. They need to know how quickly and remarkably animals respond to physical therapy. As consumers, they need to be equipped to make wise decisions and know what alternatives or adjuncts are available in veterinary care.

Knowledge is power. Animals deserve all we can give them. Enjoy the read.

Author's Note

Allow me to explain some terminology used in this book: the word "consumer" is the individual responsible for the animal's medical care and therefore the purchaser of goods and services. In my own practice, I usually refer to this person as the "client" and the animal as the "patient." In the book, I also refer to this person as the "pet owner" or "pet parent." I am aware that some prefer to use the term "pet guardian" or "caretaker." Please know that when I use the term "owner," I do not consider animals to be "chattel" or "disposable property." In fact, I feel that a pet owner belongs to their pets as much as the pets belong to their owner!

Susan E. Davis, PT

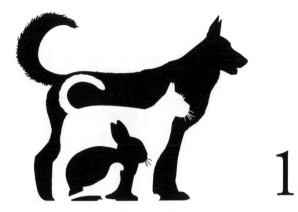

1

Emergence and Development of the Physical Therapy Field for Animals

What Is Physical Therapy?

Physical therapy (PT) dates as far back as ancient times. In the mid-400s BC, physicians such as Hippocrates began using massage and water treatments to cure afflicted individuals. By the late eighteenth century, Europe, Great Britain, and New Zealand had schools of "gymnastics" that included training in massage, movement exercises, and manual manipulations.

In the United States, physical therapy has existed in various forms since the early 1900s, when "reconstruction aides" worked in hospitals and treatment centers to help patients afflicted with polio. World Wars I and II resulted in wounded soldiers needing physical rehabilitation, which developed the foundation for the profession to grow and advance.

Modern day physical therapy is the science of applying physics and biomechanics to patients with injury, illness, loss of function, physical abnormality, and other impairments. Physical therapists study and utilize their knowledge of anatomy, physiology, kinesiology, and other sciences to evaluate and treat patients. Clinical problems are identified and likely causes determined, so that the therapist can gauge a prognosis and assessment of predicted outcome. Goals, both long and short term, are set and an intervention treatment plan is developed. Treatments consist of various exercises, functional and cognitive training, manual techniques, and physical modalities. These modalities are thermal (heat), cryo (cold), electrical, sonic (sound waves), and photo (light rays) in origin.

Physical therapists work with patients through all realms of the health care spectrum, including wellness, prevention, maintenance of fitness and health, through illness, and quality of life care. Patients from newborn through elderly receive physical therapy treatments. Physical therapists also play vital roles in education and research. (See Note 1.)

Transitioning the Field to Veterinary Medicine

Chiropractors may be the first to take credit for initially recognizing the benefits to animals of various stretching and manipulative techniques. As early as the 1920s, chiropractic school curriculums contained elements of veterinary care. In the 1960s, physical therapy began to be used in the equine field to treat athletic and thoroughbred horses in the racing and show fields. The non-invasive and effective treatments physical therapy offered were vital to helping injured horses and in preventing injury in these high-stakes arenas.

In the late 1990s, veterinarians and physical therapists began to recognize the possible benefits of physical therapy and rehabilitation to other animals, primarily canine. These included injury prevention, increased speed of physical recovery, improved quality of life, psychological benefits to the animal and owner, low risk of treatment, and reduced costs and charges. The American Physical Therapy Association (APTA) and American Veterinary Medicine Association (AVMA) began mutual communication and collaboration to develop position statements and identify guidelines for areas of animal practice. The first education programs for animal physical therapy appeared in 2000 and 2001, offered at veterinary schools to licensed veterinarians, physical therapists, physical therapist assistants, and veterinary technicians. The University of Tennessee, Knoxville, was the first to develop programs in post-graduate training for equine and canine rehabilitation. Because the use of the term "physical therapy" is protected in many states, meaning that it can only be used when licensed physical therapists perform the service, the new term "canine rehabilitation" was coined.

In recent years, the use of physical therapy and rehabilitation for animals has expanded from use in equine and canine fields to include felines, farm animals, exotics such as avian, reptiles, and so on. For the purposes of this book, my primary focus will be on canine, but I mention other animal applications in various sections. I love interacting with as many species as possible and find unique joys in working with each. Cats, for example, are generally assumed to be uncooperative with therapy but most do not resist the hands-on part and actively enjoy exercise involving balls, rocker boards, climbing, games, etc. Birds are surprisingly tolerant with handling and are keen observers of a therapist's every move. I marvel at their intellect! Rabbits are sweet, but oh so delicate and require special care. Monkeys enjoy physical therapy, especially "grooming" the therapist, picking lint off jackets, and rearranging hair. Goats are charming and fun to be with, though their span of patience is limited. Guinea pigs make cute, interesting sounds and nibble away while you work with them. Speaking of swine, potbelly pigs make fun, curious patients, especially if you can work as they try to nose-root for whatever is in your pockets. Camels can be friendly too and love massage and manual joint mobilizations, as long as the therapist doesn't mind using a stepladder. The large and growing field of equine physical therapy and rehabilitation will not be included in this book, as it has developed into its own highly specialized field requiring a separate education and training tract for physical therapists.

What physical therapy for animals is NOT: It is not and should never be used as a substitute for primary veterinary care. Physical therapy is instead an adjunct to or an ancillary part of primary veterinary care. The best practice is to provide physical therapy concurrently with veterinary care, along with good communication. Physical therapists cannot prescribe medications or give advice about vaccinations, surgery, or any medical care that a licensed doctor of veterinary medicine has the education and authority to perform. A competent physical therapist will know her limits and refer all questions about primary medicine to the veterinarian. Physical therapy should never be used as a substitute for medication, unless an animal is unable to take medicines and needs PT for pain and other symptom relief. Physical therapy can be given in conjunction with medications prescribed by a veterinarian in therapeutic or as-needed dosing instructions. In some cases, as the animal improves with physical therapy, medications can be weaned and even discontinued, per a veterinarian's advice.

Physical therapists are not animal trainers or behaviorists. Physical therapists are educated in basic training commands, handling, animal restraint, and general animal behavior, but can only utilize these skills or answer questions as these areas apply directly to rehabilitation treatment. The physical therapist should be able to recommend qualified veterinarians, animal trainers, and behaviorists in your geographic area for any needed referrals.

Traditional versus Holistic

You may be wondering where PT and rehabilitation for your pet fits in the veterinary paradigm: is it holistic or traditional? On one of my first marketing missions to an animal hospital, after introducing myself and my services, I met a veterinarian who said, "Sorry, but I don't favor the use of holistic practices for my patients." Shocked, I said, "Holistic? This is physical therapy!" In that particular encounter, I was unsuccessful in my attempt to explain the true nature of animal PT. In human medicine, PT is very much a part of traditional Western health care. It is an adjunct to other aspects of medicine such as pre- and post-surgery, during chemotherapy, dialysis, with medications, and so on. It is very similar in veterinary care, but usually called "complementary." Many pet parents likely think of PT as "alternative" or "holistic" because it is a non-chemical form of treatment, but it is definitely traditional and not meant to be different from conventional veterinary care. However, aspects of holistic or Eastern medicine, such as Reiki or acupressure, blend beautifully with PT and can be incorporated into treatment. Physical therapists are not at all against holistic practices, we are just not fundamentally trained that way. One of the first weeks I began providing PT at a shelter, a kennel attendant told me I had "awesome energy" in my hands. I thought she meant that I had strong and sturdy fingers! Of course, I now understand that she was referring to biofield energy, which I have come to appreciate over the past few years, working alongside Reiki practitioners, energy healers, and animal communicators.

Qualifications

Exiting the practice of physical therapy for people after thirty-one years and entering the field of veterinary physical rehabilitation in 2008 was a huge career transition. I entered a world where what I did was no longer called physical therapy and many of the providers were not actual physical therapists. Most canine rehabilitation practitioners are vets and veterinary technicians who have taken courses and certification programs to learn the various modalities, exercises, and manual skills needed to help animals recover from injury, surgery, and illness. As previously mentioned, the term "physical therapy" is protected and used only when patient care is rendered by a licensed physical therapist. So, is there a difference in canine physical rehabilitation and canine physical therapy? They are inherently the same service, provided by different professionals. I should note that some physical therapists have a dual designation of PT and CCRP (certified canine rehabilitation practitioner). For the pet owner, what is important is that the person working with your animal is a qualified medical professional with extensive additional training. For example, the provider should be a veterinarian or veterinary technician with training in physical rehabilitation, or a licensed physical therapist with training in animal anatomy, pathology, and related veterinary topics. It should not be a physical therapy aide or a vet receptionist who is simply office-trained in putting your pet in a water treadmill tank. This field requires a solid medical background, knowledge of gait mechanics, muscle and joint function, and a high level of skill in manual techniques and physical modalities.

As more physical therapists become trained to work with animals, you will see a trend toward the field being called "physical therapy for animals," rather than "canine rehabilitation." Other forms of treatment, such as chiropractic and massage therapy, can also benefit your pet. These are related to the rehabilitation field, but are generally not substitutes for it, and should only be provided by those with cross-training experience in animals. (Please note this perspective is from the United States; other countries may have different practice patterns.)

BEST GUIDANCE
In most states in the country, "physical therapy" is a protected term and can be used only if the person performing treatment is a licensed physical therapist. It is not a generic term. If your pet's service is being provided by a vet or other non-physical therapist, it should be called "rehabilitation."

Practice Settings

Animal physical therapy and rehabilitation is predominantly provided in veterinary offices or hospitals and clinic settings. An alternative practice model can occur in the animal patient's private home or other location, which might be an animal shelter, kennel, zoo, wildlife refuge, aquarium, farm, or sanctuary. I admit to having a personal bias to home care—both foster and forever homes—and my hope is that this will become more available in the future as the field grows. There is a distinct advantage in giving care where the pet feels most relaxed and comfortable. The down side of this is if a pet needs use of large equipment, such as underwater treadmills, agility courses, or use of large, non-portable equipment. In these cases, the home-based or mobile therapist should refer you to a facility that provides this type of service.

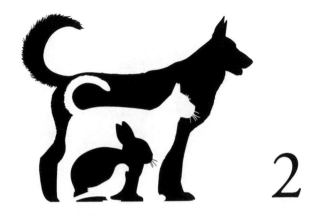

2

Getting Started and the First Visit

Choosing a Therapist

Finding the right physical therapy practitioner for your pet is important, but not daunting, if you consider your needs in advance of the initial contact. After ensuring the provider is qualified, factors such as location, availability, and cost are usually considered next. Your decision may be based on whether you can transport your pet practically, what type of services and equipment will be needed, and so on. The first step is to gather information about what is available in your area—through the Internet, word of mouth, phone directories, and referrals from your veterinarian—and then begin contacting the service providers. Therapists, veterinarians, and their staff members should be willing to answer your questions by phone, email, Skype, or in person, to help you make an informed decision. It is not unreasonable to expect a practitioner to spend ten to fifteen minutes with you. Ask to take a brief tour of the facility, unless a video tour is available online.

Initial Evaluation

Your pet's initial visit is usually scheduled within a few days of contact, unless there is a reason for a waiting period based on your veterinarian's instruction (e.g., healing of a surgical incision). It will typically last an hour and consist of an evaluation along with home instructions. Optimally, the therapist will include some treatment as well in that visit. If treatment is recommended before an evaluation has been performed, you should not use that provider.

Here's how the evaluation typically goes:

The therapist should always start out by greeting your pet. Don't be shocked if the therapist actually introduces herself by name to the pet and explains that she is here to provide physical therapy and help, etc. I do this routinely and both the animal and its owner seem to appreciate it! Some practitioners with Eastern medical backgrounds believe that one should ask permission of the animal before beginning any evaluation or procedure. Though I'm not sure how you receive an answer, I've been told that as long as the animal does not give a signal of rejection, you have received sufficient permission. I confess to

BEST GUIDANCE
Every state in the country has laws and regulations governing the practice of physical therapy. Many states have direct access, enabling you to go directly to a physical therapist for care. In providing physical therapy for animals, a collaborative care model is best. That includes seeing your veterinarian for a health review and medical clearance prior to initiating physical therapy.

not going to that extreme in my daily practice, but the greeting and introduction should definitely be included.

You will be asked to fill out a history form or provide verbal and written information of past medical and health issues, medications taken, types and dates of surgery, etc. The therapist will then start the examination consisting of the following areas:

Appearance and Posture: The therapist will examine weight distribution between fore and hind limbs, looking at the topline of the body to determine if it is normal for the breed. For example, a normal topline for a German Shepherd is one that slopes downward toward the tail. A topline that shows "roaching," or is curved upward and rounded, is abnormal in most breeds.

Palpation: By using hands and fingers, the therapist will feel various structures, such as muscles, tendons, bones, and other tissue for any abnormalities. Temperature, swelling, degree of hardness or softness in the muscle and soft tissue, tone and alignment of the structures can provide the therapist useful information.

Measurements: Tape measures, rulers, and other devices such as goniometers are used to document baseline limb lengths, circumference around the limb, height and length, and degrees of motion. If one limb is being treated due to surgery, the other normal limb should also be measured in order to compare the differences. Normative charts are also available to the practitioner to help establish degrees of abnormality. Range of motion will be measured at the various joints to determine the amount of flexion, extension, rotation, abduction, and adduction the pet has, and these figures will be documented in the record and compared to other joints in your pet's body along with established normal values. All of these baseline values will be used to track your pet's progress, as remeasurements are taken during the course of treatment.

End Feel: As the therapist moves joints and limbs through their range of motion, various tensions and responses will be detected, especially at the end of the range, called "end feel." Terms the therapist might use for end feel are taut, leathery, capsular, springy, soft, blocked, guarded, or empty.

Strength: Various manual techniques and some mechanical devices can be used to determine muscle strength. This is usually graded on a scale of zero to five, with five being normal. Other therapists use a grading scale of normal, good, fair, poor, trace, and zero.

Function: Basic activities of daily living are measured, such as grooming, eating, bowel and bladder duties, moving from sitting to standing and reverse, climbing up/down steps, lying down and getting up from bed, as well as the ability to play with toys and interact with other pets or family members. The therapist will assign scores of independent, maximum assistance, moderate assistance, minimal assistance, close contact guarding, or supervision, to describe how your pet performs these duties.

Walking: Also called "ambulation." The therapist will look at how independent your pet can walk on its own, or whether your pet needs assistance with a cart or sling, or needs to be carried.

The amount of weight the pet places on its limbs, or weight bearing, is observed and graded as full, partial, toe-touch, or non-weight bearing. Next is determining the distance or duration that the pet can walk, measured in feet, meters, miles, time, etc. These factors are estimated by either keen observation or use of scales, pedometers, or kinetic devices using force plates that capture ground reaction forces.

The final area is that of gait deviations, requiring professional observation and experience. These nuances or patterns of walking provide valuable clues to what is happening in the neurological, muscular, and skeletal system. Here are some examples of gait deviations that you and the therapist may observe:

> Head Bobbing: The animal's head literally bobs up and down during each step, in an overexaggerated style. This usually indicates pain on stepping. The excessive head and neck movement is an attempt to take weight off the painful weight bearing.

> Knuckling: The animal's paw or paws will curl under with the toes tucked beneath, resulting in rolling over onto the knuckles, instead of landing flat on the toe pads. Knuckling usually indicates weakness, primarily from the spine and spinal nerves.

> Antalgia, or Limping: Describes when the animal lifts the limb up off the ground too early in the cycle, thereby favoring it. It also means that the animal is spending less time on that limb in the stance phase of the cycle. Antalgia is an indication of pain.

Floating Gait: Is observed when the forelimbs move in an irregular high step or prancing fashion, and the front of the body looks like it is lifting off or floating above the ground. This can indicate instability in the neck or neurological problems.

Ataxia, or Drunken Gait: Shows the animal staggering or moving clumsily, unable to balance or control its movements. This can indicate problems of a neurological nature in the brain or spinal cord, as well as vestibular problems from the ear.

Many other deviations, such as dragging of limbs, parts being held too stiffly, joints showing excessive laxity or instability, turning outward or inward to an abnormal degree, along with countless others, can be valuable indicators to help you, the therapist, and the veterinarian determine how to help your pet.

Scoring: Overall scores of lameness and function can be used to summarize your pet's status for quick reference. Being familiar with these scores can help you, your therapist, and veterinarian communicate and establish baseline values and chart ongoing progress. Here are the values:

Lameness Score at a Walk
  0 Walks normally, deviations are absent, full weight bearing on all strides observed
  1 Walks with slight lameness, deviations are minor, partial weight bearing
  2 Obvious lameness, partial to toe-touch weight bearing

3 Severe lameness, intermittent toe-touch weight bearing

4 Full lameness, non-weight bearing, may be unable to stand (See Note 2.)

Neurologic Scale for Movement and Walking

5 Normal strength and coordination

4 Can stand on own; minimal weakness and loss of coordination

3 Can stand on own but frequently stumbles and falls; mild weakness and loss of coordination

2 Unable to stand without support, needs assistance, moves limbs readily but stumbles and falls frequently; moderate weakness and loss of coordination

1 Unable to stand without full assistance, moves limbs slightly; severe weakness and loss of coordination

0 Absence of purposeful movement, paralysis

BEST GUIDANCE
Never skip or marginalize the importance of the initial evaluation, as it is a critical component to your pet's care and provides the foundation for clinical decisions.

You may have noticed that the Lameness Scale at Walking test's best score is 0, while the Neurological test's best score is 5. While I wish the tests' scores were consistent in using high numbers to represent the healthiest and zero as most in need, unfortunately they are not.

Functional Scale

There is also a canine Functional Scale that measures ability to run, jump, climb, roll, stand, get up and down from lying, urinate and defecate, on a 1 to 5 scale. Overall score will be best out of a possible score of seventy.

Balance: This is tested in the sitting and standing positions. Static balance is the ability of the animal to keep its balance without any external disturbances. Dynamic balance is the ability of the animal to maintain its balance while the therapist manually pushes against or resists it. The therapist should use a gentle push. Grading of balance is documented as excellent, fair, poor, and absent. A fair grade means that the animal starts to lose its balance easily but can regain it on its own. Poor grades indicate that the animal loses balance easily and can't regain it.

Neurological Testing: Typically, the therapist will do neurological testing if she suspects problems in this area. Suspicions of neurological involvement occur with problems of controlling bowel and bladder, gradual onset of lameness, balance difficulties, etc. In these cases, the evaluation will include neurological tests of reflexes and sensation. The therapist will text reflexes with a rubber hammer or her fingers at the toes, knee/stifle, elbow/biceps, and other locations. Responses to reflex testing can be normal, exaggerated, or absent. A quick, brisk response is normal. Exaggerated responses are large in scope and sustained. Weaker or lack of response is abnormal. A brush or other utensil can be used in a stroking or sweeping motion along the flank to elicit a muscle twitch, testing the spinal reflexes. There are other reaction tests involving placing the paw in an abnormal weight-bearing position and seeing if the animal can self-correct it. Gently squeezing or pinching between the toes or at the paw should elicit a pulling away response. This is sometimes called "flexor withdrawal."

Reflexive motor tone in the muscles can be tested by the therapist performing certain movements of the pet's joints. Tone is labeled as normal, hyper-reflexive or spastic, and hypo-reflexive or flaccid.

Sensation and pain can be difficult to evaluate in an animal, as it cannot verbally describe symptoms as a human being can. A numb area can sometimes be identified by the pet excessively licking or biting it. The animal will also try to shake the limb in an attempt to change the sensation. Pain can be demonstrated in many species by crying or whimpering, decreased eating, moving slowly, trembling, panting, refusal to make eye-to-eye contact, a rounded or hunched posture (or roaching), and even nipping or biting.

Setting Goals

What do we want to accomplish? What is the final outcome we wish to achieve?

Goals are often what keep us going through life, striving to attain our dreams. I can assure you that your pet has built-in goals and always seeks to reach them through its natural survival instincts. For human beings in the role of doctor, therapist, guardian, or caregiver, structured and documented goals form the framework of achieving success for the animal. Goals should be documented, mutually agreed upon by all parties, and revisited regularly. Animals are likely to make the greatest gains when therapy focuses on the goals set during the initial visit.

BEST GUIDANCE
Your therapist should apply this philosophy to your pet's care: "Man is a goal-seeking animal. His life only has meaning if he is reaching out and striving for his goals." —Aristotle

When the evaluation is complete, the therapist reviews the findings and makes a list of problems from the deficit areas. From this list, long- and short-term goals can be formulated to work toward achieving them. The therapist should include you in the goal-setting process by asking you what your perceptions are, what you would like the pet to be able to achieve, what seems realistic, etc. Your answer might be, "I'd like my cat to be able to jump from her perch or platform without falling and hitting her head when she lands." Other responses might include wanting a pet to be able to groom herself, return to working or herding activities, climb steps in and out of the home, and so on. Goals will be set based on your opinions, what the therapist observes during the evaluation, his/her professional experience, and documented clinical information on available outcomes. Sometimes a physical therapist may think the pet owner's desired outcome is unreasonable or not achievable based on the evaluation findings. A true and honest discussion should take place so that both parties understand each other and know what goals are reasonable.

Short-term goals consist of the areas that must be met in order for the global long-term goals to be achieved. An example of a long-term goal is "leash walking for one mile in twenty minutes, with zero or minimal gait deviations." Corresponding short-term goals to aid in meeting this long-term goal might be "increase strength of hind limbs to a grade of good"; "improve coordination of limb placement"; "achieve normal range of motion of the stifle/knee," and so on. These should be as specific and measureable as possible.

The overall goals should contain the following elements: who, what, under what circumstances, how well, and by when. "Who" refers to the patient, although the owner and family members, and even other pets in the household, are considered. "What" refers to the activity the patient will perform. "Under what circumstances" is the component of the goal that is the condition under which the patient's achievement is measured. "How well" describes the amount of assistance required or the quality of how the task is performed. "By when" is the target date for the patient to achieve the goal. Putting it all together, a complete goal should look something like this: "Fido will go for walks with the family, with a harness and lead, with partial to full weight bearing, on pavement, grass, and uneven terrain, for twenty to thirty minutes daily, without limping or knuckling of the affected limb, by eight weeks post-surgery."

Precautions and Contraindications

Your therapist is responsible for knowing what precautions need to be taken in any clinical situation and informing you of these. However, it is reasonable and advised that you as the pet owner ask about potential precautions. There are also contraindications that the therapist must be aware of and identify, so that your pet is not harmed.

Examples of precautions are:

- Use a muzzle if there is a risk of the animal biting.
- Wear gloves or apply a plastic clear barrier to avoid direct contact with an open wound.
- Shield the animal's eyes if a certain type of laser is used.
- Apply a gentler-than-normal pressure during massage or joint mobilization if a pain response is present.
- Make the therapist immediately aware if your dog has/ is being treated for kennel cough or if your cat has an upper respiratory infection. It must be isolated from other pets to avoid contamination or scheduled at the end of the day. If the therapist has provided treatment to another contagious animal, request that she change clothes or cover with a clean scrub top or lab coat.

Each individual animal has its own threshold for pain or tolerance of treatment. The therapist and pet owner must continuously monitor for any changes in behavior that could signal an aggressive or fear response. The therapist should have a policy on when and how to use restraint, head halters, or muzzles. Warning signs to look for include growling, refusal of the animal to make direct eye contact, ears in retracted position, tail downward, and elevation of hair or fur along the spine. If any of these signs are identified, expect the therapist to require that the animal be muzzled. Many types and sizes of muzzles exist, so you might be asked to provide a suitable type for your pet. Most therapists will have a set available, such as the Mikki muzzle in various sizes. There are leather types, those made of mesh, and the larger basket muzzle as well. The muzzle should be used for the shortest time possible, with verbal reassurances given to the pet during use. The pet should be rewarded with a treat immediately upon removal of the muzzle. If the therapist asks to use a muzzle on your pet, it is best to comply with this and not refuse. The therapist has the right to refuse to provide treatment in turn. If your care provider is bitten and requires medical treatment, she will probably need to report the incident to local authorities to comply with state statutes. Everyone wants to avoid this, so both parties need to be aware of warning signs and take prudent precautions.

Contraindications are specific reasons not to do something, or situations where something cannot be done or used because it is dangerous or harmful. Contraindications can be absolute but other times are relative. In the latter, the pros and cons must be weighed against each other. The contraindication becomes relative to the risks versus the benefits.

Examples of contraindications are:

- Using laser directly on the eyes, over a growth plate in the bone of a young animal.
- Applying laser or ultrasound over a cancerous tumor.
- Performing vigorous exercise during an active infection.
- Mobilizing an already unstable joint.

A relative contraindication may be reversed, when the benefits outweigh the risks. For example, laser might be used over a bone fracture site near or over a growth plate if there is a high probability that, without it, the fracture wouldn't heal well and the limb would likely be amputated. In that case, it would be better to risk the possibility of partially stunted growth, and spare the limb.

Finally, there is the "something just doesn't seem right" scenario, where extra caution must be applied. An experienced therapist should possess a sixth sense that prompts a warning signal to delay initiation of treatment or stop ongoing care, along with appropriate recommendations to the pet owner.

Here is an example of such a situation I encountered in early 2012:

Mrs. Angela S contacted me about setting up physical therapy for her ten-year-old male Cattle Dog/Border Collie mix named Scout, who was dragging one of the hind limbs. I asked her several questions over the phone and began to feel some concern when the symptoms and signs Scout was displaying didn't seem typical. In addition, when I asked about the veterinarian's work-up to date, it was fairly minimal with only an office exam and recommendation to "try some physical therapy." I explained that I did not feel comfortable initiating the physical therapy process until Scout had more testing and a definitive diagnosis established, or that other serious conditions be ruled out first. I offered a few suggestions, then we hung up. I made some notes about our conversation in case she called back at a future date, but I didn't hear from her.

In early March, I received the following email from Angela:

Dear Susan, A few weeks ago I called you about my dog Scout. He was having trouble walking and the doctor has suggested that PT might help. You were kind enough to discuss some options with me. Tonight, I am writing to say "thank you," for your wonderful advice. You suggested that

I return to the vet and ask about having some X-rays done and you also recommended a specialty veterinary hospital for additional opinions. That is where Scout has been receiving treatment for cancer since February. Unfortunately it was discovered that Scout had a large tumor on his skull. A neuro-surgeon removed it and he is recovering, along with radiation treatment. He is expected to do well with his recovery. Thank you again for your find and professional advice. Without it, Scout and our family might not have had this happy ending.

You can imagine my shock, but also relief, that I had not initiated physical therapy and potentially delayed finding a tumor once it was too late.

Assessment

The assessment process is where true analysis comes in to play. Clinical judgments are made based on the information gained in the evaluation. The following questions need to be asked and answered by the therapist: "What's wrong here?" "What type of tissue is involved?" "What is causing this to happen?" Is this the same thing as making a diagnosis? No. The medical diagnosis comes from the primary veterinarian, unless your therapist is a rehabilitation-trained veterinarian. For example, a global diagnosis of degenerative myelopathy or ligament sprain will usually be established by the veterinarian before you see the physical therapist. The physical therapist will then thoroughly assess all of the underlying specific mechanisms causing your pet's problems (sometimes called a "PT diagnosis"), before the treatment plan is made. The veterinarian's diagnosis is the macro portion of the process, followed by the therapist's micro analysis. Breaking down each problem and determining causative factors, as close as possible, will ensure that the treatment will specifically address your pet's needs. It will also help the therapist directly focus treatment toward attaining the targeted goals set in the evaluation. Treatment will be more efficient, with greater outcomes and faster results when an assessment is carefully made.

If this sounds complicated and time-consuming, I can assure you that an experienced clinician can make assessments in a relatively quick time frame. Even the most complex and challenging cases can usually be assessed in a few minutes, after reviewing all of the evaluation findings.

Prognosis

The prognosis is a prediction of the level of improvement your pet will ultimately achieve. It includes how well the therapist expects your pet to fare with treatment, how likely the pet is to achieve the set of goals, and more. Essentially, it defines the potential for recovery. Prognosis is typically graded as excellent, good, fair, or poor. It should be discussed frankly with you, the pet's owner. Along with this should be an estimate of the length of time needed to achieve the goals. This can be quantified in terms of weeks, or occasionally months. A good clinician can generally predict how your pet will likely respond to treatment: fast, medium, or slow.

Treatment Plan and Intervention

Next the therapist will formulate a plan of intervention, or treatment to help your pet succeed and meet the goals that have been set. The treatment plan should be put in writing as part of the pet's medical record. A typical physical therapy treatment plan will include the following areas: physical modalities, manual or hands-on techniques, therapeutic exercises, functional activities, gait training, and home instruction. Treatment may also include wound care, first aid, bandaging, assisting with the administration of medications, measuring for assistive devices, or providing advice and education that can benefit the animal, mirroring the goals. Any procedure or method of treatment provided to your pet should be explained to you in a manner that you can fully understand. All care provided by a physical therapist can be done in full view of the pet owner and nothing should be "taken to the back room" of a facility.

In deciding what methods to use in treatment, the therapist will consider the following questions: Is the condition acute, sub-acute, or chronic? Can the animal tolerate a normal amount of pressure or intensity of exercise, or must I modify techniques to accommodate special needs? Which physical modalities are best suited for the type of condition presented? What are the most effective exercises for this type of injury? Treatment plans are not a one-size-fits-all recipe, but must be individually tailored for each animal. Even when a therapist has been

BEST GUIDANCE
The best treatment intervention plans are those that allow the entire team to communicate together, including the pet.

provided with a veterinary surgeon's protocol to follow, flexibility and professional judgments supersede in order to accommodate unique traits or needs.

Conditions heal at different rates depending on various factors such as the type of tissue that had been injured, and what stage of recovery it is currently in. The first is the acute stage, which is early after the injury, when inflammation is present, along with swelling, sharp pain, redness, irritation, and often a feeling of heat when touching the area. Range of motion is usually painful and limited. The animal may yelp when the area is palpated quickly or with too much pressure, as tissue sensitivity may be high. This phase begins within the initial moments after injury and lasts about five to seven days.

The next phase, called sub-acute, is characterized by decreasing signs of inflammation and swelling, with a normalized tissue temperature. Pain can still be present, but more of a dull than sharp nature. You will be able to touch the injured area without eliciting a painful response from the animal. Mobility and range of motion will still be limited, but not to as great an extent as in the acute phase. In this phase, new blood capillaries, collagen, and granular tissue begin to form. This stage usually lasts two to six weeks.

The chronic stage of healing involves final remodeling and alignment of tissues, as the healing ends and recovery matures. Inflammation is fully resolved at this point and tissues are nearly free of pain when pressure is applied. Range of motion will be increased, but typically with some pain and tightness at the ends of the range. As tissue heals, the body often overcompensates by extra remodeling, scar tissue formation, and adhesions, which can cause tightness and spasms. The chronic phase begins after six weeks and may last six months up to one year. If a condition is still present after one year, it is considered long term in its chronicity. This does not mean that it is permanent or will never heal, but that interventions are needed to break the cycle and achieve full resolution of symptoms.

All of these factors will be considered when final decisions are made in the treatment plan. A good therapist should use variety in providing treatment and be able to adapt to conditions as they change. She should possess multiple ways and techniques to accomplish a desired effect and have a limitless bag of tricks from which to draw. As a pet owner, you should feel confident that the therapist loves what she does and has the talent needed to produce results.

Are you wondering if animals like having physical therapy treatments? The answer is yes! At first, they might not be exactly sure what is going on, but in a very short amount of time they figure it out and like the experience. I had one patient a few years ago at an animal shelter, a lively Weimaraner named Chloe, who liked having therapy so much that she faked limping to get my attention! Chloe had treatments for about a month after an injury to her elbow sustained through rough play with another dog. After six visits she was symptom-free and no longer showed any lameness, so I discharged her. Well, she figured out a way to get back on my clinic schedule by suddenly limping when she saw me in the building. At first I thought the kennel attendants were teasing me, but they insisted I observe Chloe from a distance, hidden behind a shed, and I saw her playing and running in the yard in perfect form. As soon as I got closer and she spotted me, the limp started to dramatically appear. I gave her the nickname "Academy Award Actress" and always found a few spare minutes at the end of the day to give her some attention and massage.

Like Chloe, your pet should enjoy the treatment sessions and be rewarded with lots of praise, treats, or other positive reinforcements from the therapist. The therapist should be consistent in her standard of treatment, delivery, and demeanor. You and your pet should never wonder what mood the therapist is in today or what her caseload is like. A true professional will leave her personal baggage at the door and maintain a cheerful, positive outlook at all times. Here is where I admit to being a bit "old school" but I firmly believe that during treatment therapists should never talk about anything in her personal life, unless the pet owner specifically asks. Any discussions that include potentially unpleasant or sad feelings should be discontinued or avoided, as the animal will instantly pick up on this. If the animal feels stress or the need to protect the therapist, the impact of treatment will be diminished. My motto is "It's never about me, and it's all about the pets!"

Your pet should be positioned comfortably during therapy, with special pillows, beanbags, rolls, or bolsters placed to support the area of the body being treated. All special needs should be fully accommodated: If a large dog feels more comfortable staying in its crate, the therapist can reach inside or even crawl into the crate with the dog for part of the treatment, if necessary. Short rest periods should be interspersed throughout the session, especially during the acute phase, and the pet should be given a chew treat or a simple "time out," while the therapist makes chart notes, discusses treatment response, or answers your questions.

Are you wondering if therapy will be painful? The answer is no! All aspects of therapy treatment can be administered in a careful, soothing, gentle manner. Your pet may experience mild discomfort at times, but nothing should be harsh or considered painful for the animal. Your pet might be tired and sleep a lot after the first treatment session, but it should not be unduly sore afterward. The therapist will tell you what to expect. There may be some soreness present, but it should not last more than a few hours after the initial treatment. If your pet is sore for an entire day or more, then the treatment was probably too aggressive and will need to be modified.

If you do not see any improvement after the first visit, don't be disappointed. It usually takes two or three visits for a noticeable response to occur. Sometimes, however, you will see a marked improvement right away. If there is no improvement at all after three visits, the therapist should modify the treatment plan and move onto Plan B. If the animal shows any adverse response to care or becomes worse, treatment should be discontinued and the veterinarian notified immediately. Physical therapy is not an exact science, and it is impossible to predict every scenario, but your therapist should base her care on best practices in the industry and prudent thinking. Although very rare, mistakes can be made and your therapist should be open, honest, and accountable in all situations.

A final word about treatment intervention is that of owner compliance. You have hired the physical therapist to do a job, but you, as the pet owner, need to put your faith and trust in the clinician and follow her instructions as closely as possible. If you are given instructions that seem unrealistic to carry out based on your work schedule, tell the therapist so that modifications can be made. On the other hand, don't assume that if "five repetitions is good, then ten is better." Your dedication and enthusiasm might cause you to over-exercise the pet and result in swelling, pain, and lameness.

The best treatment intervention plans are those in which the whole team—therapist, veterinarian, pet owner, and pet patient—works and communicates together!

Basic Anatomy

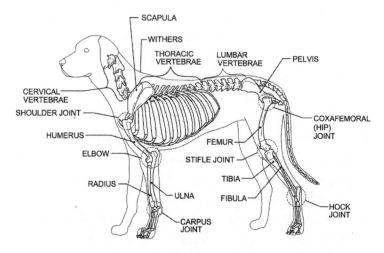

Figure 1

Let's take a look at the basic structural anatomy of animals in order to have a frame of reference for the sections to come. Although this illustration shows a dog, it represents the anatomy of most all animal species that are quadrupeds, or walking on four legs.

Starting at the head, the vertebrae of the neck, called "cervical vertebrae," are stacked, with discs in between, and allow support and movement of the head. Next is the forelimb, consisting of a shoulder blade, called "scapula," and joints—shoulder, elbow, and carpus (like our wrist). The shoulder is a ball-and-socket joint, formed by the caved, curved end of the scapula and the ball or head of the long humerus bone.

The middle joint is the elbow, formed by the distal end of the humerus and the radius and ulna bones. The radius and ulna form the ante brachium, which is similar to the human forearm. Below this is the carpus joint, similar to the human wrist. The carpus is formed by the distal ends of the radius and ulna and the small carpal bones, long metacarpal bones of the paw, and finally, the phalanx bones, which form the digits (similar to fingers) of the forepaw. I find the easiest way to visualize these joints is to ask a client to get on the floor on his or her hands and knees. The client's arms are now essentially like the animal's forelimb, complete with shoulder, elbow, wrist, etc. Of course, the joints are built a bit differently to handle weight bearing in the animal. The animal's shoulder socket is shallower and less developed than a human's, with the joint capsule and surrounding muscles providing the bulk of support. There is no significant clavicle or collar bone in dogs and other animals, compared to humans. Whereas the human arm is designed for mobility, the quadruped animal's "arm" or forelimb is designed for stability and weight bearing.

Moving along the body is the spine, running parallel to the ground. First are the thoracic vertebrae and ribs, forming the chest and middle section of the spine. Next are the lumbar vertebrae, similar to the lower back of a human. The lumbar vertebrae attach to the pelvis and continue to form a chain of small bones into the tail. In the hind limb, the first joint is the hip, or coxofemoral joint, formed by the pelvic socket and the round head of the long femur bone. The animal pelvis tends to be narrower than a human being's, with the hip joint designed more for motion and propulsion than for bearing weight. The thigh continues along the femur, coming to the middle joint called the stifle, similar to the human knee. The stifle is formed by the distal end of the femur and the tibia and fibula. The tibia and fibula form the leg, continuing to the hock joint, similar to the human ankle. This is also referred to as the tarsus joint. The hock is formed by the distal ends of the tibia and fibula, and the calcaneus bone of the heel, talus, and tarsal bones, then finally the long metatarsal bones and small phalanx bones of the digits, or toes. The hind paw consists of these last mentioned bones and is referred to as the rear pastern. You might have noticed that animals stand on their toes and do not bear weight on the heels. This allows them the angulation and mechanics needed to jump and run efficiently. It is understandable that clients often ask why their pets' knees bend backward, and I have to repress a grin as I explain that it is not a knee, but actually a heel.

For animal species that are bipedal and stand on two limbs, such as birds, apes, kangaroos, and some lizards, the anatomy is quite similar. Their lower limbs contain the same major bones as the hind limbs of the dog, cat, or other quadruped animal. Birds have a different number of vertebrae, especially in the cervical or neck region. The bird's beautiful feathered wings share the same bones (scapula, humerus, radius, ulna) and joints (shoulder, elbow, carpus) of the canine forelimb. The avian bones are much lighter to allow for flight and the digits or "fingers" are formed uniquely for the attachment of various sizes and shapes of feathers, or coverts.

Muscles, tendons, and ligaments in animals are similar to that of humans. Major muscles that may sound familiar to the reader, such as biceps, triceps, hamstrings, quadriceps, gluteal, and lats, are also present in animals, serving the same basic functions.

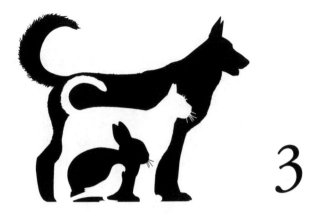

3

Treatment Using Physical Modalities

Laser

It's time to explore "Photon Power!" The word "laser" is an acronym for light amplification by stimulated emission of radiation. It is emitted through an LED, or light emitting diode.

Lasers are one of the most underutilized treatment modalities that we have to offer animals in the veterinary world. Yet it is one of the safest and most effective devices to utilize. As more animal physical therapists and veterinarians use laser in animal treatment, it will increase in popularity and availability in clinics and other forms of practice.

A laser generates a beam of very intense light. The term "cold laser" simply means that the light is subthermal and penetrates the skin with no heating effect or damage to the skin. To have an understanding of how it works you have to go back to the basic form of all matter: the atom. The atom consists of protons, neutrons, and electrons moving around a nucleus. When an electromagnetic charge is applied, electrons change orbits and photons are released. Photons are bundles of energy that carry light to the body. During everyday life, photons from ordinary and man-made light bombard the skin's surface but do not penetrate beyond the surface of the skin. Laser has certain properties having to do with its color and polarization that allow it to penetrate the skin and be absorbed into the tissues below.

When the light, in the form of photons, reaches the tissues below, it directs energy to the body's cells, which the cells then convert into chemical energy. So basically it starts with physics and ends with chemistry! Photons, absorbed into the cell membranes, trigger biological changes within the body and kick-off cellular energy systems (remember the Krebs cycle from biology class?).

Photons will only be absorbed by the cells that have been injured and need help. The result is increased healing, decreased pain, reduction of unwanted scar tissue, decreased bacterial counts, reduced inflammation, etc. In some cases, it can actually help accelerate the formation of good scar tissue. Laser therapy does not just speed up healing, it actually improves repair, regeneration, and remodeling of tissue.

Therefore, laser is usually very effective in the following conditions: hip and elbow dysplasia, arthritis, muscle strains, ligament sprains, post-surgery to seal incisions, skin conditions such as ulcerations, open wounds, lick granulomas, and to speed up healing of fractures. There is also emerging evidence of its use in nerve regeneration and spinal cord injuries.

Laser procedure is painless and fast. It sometimes requires shaving the animal's coat if very thick and long, covering the animal's eyes, or using protective gear, depending on the type of equipment used. It usually elicits a brief high-pitched signal, to alert the user of the instant the laser begins. Laser is given to your pet via a probe or pad. If using it directly over a wound or open incision, the therapist should sanitize the probe or pad and apply a clear plastic barrier first. Delivered in joules of light, the most powerful laser units deliver 1 joule in one to five seconds. Dosage is determined by the body part, the overall body size, and color of the animal's coat.

Laser units have two key parameters that dictate their function or capability: wavelength, measured in nanometers, and power, measured in milliwatts. True laser starts at wavelength of 800nm (anything lower than that is considered to be infrared light) and power of 500 to 900 milliwatts. Be careful if you are tempted to purchase home models that advertise having high wavelengths of 600, 770, or even 800 nm. It sounds good but usually the power is so low that they are not very effective or able to elicit a measurable clinical response. Wavelength alone is not effective without sufficient power.

Laser should not be used for animals that are sensitive to light, over a cancerous tumor, in or near the eyes, during pregnancy, directly over growth plates, during an active infection, or when antibiotics or high levels of steroids have just been started. Sometimes the vet or physical therapist may have to weigh the benefits versus the risks when deciding to use laser in unique situations; I recently had to decide to use laser over a growth plate for a compound fracture in the shoulder of a Terrier mix that would have resulted in probable limb amputation. In that case, the risk of having laser affect the growth plate was less important than the attempt to save the limb. I am happy to say that we (the vet and I) made the right decision as the fracture was healed quickly with laser and the limb preserved, with no apparent loss of length.

The pet owner should feel at liberty to ask important questions when laser treatment is used. It should be performed by a veterinarian, an animal-trained physical therapist, or an animal-trained chiropractor. You can ask about the laser's power and wavelength. If the provider does not know, or is unwilling to tell you, then beware that the unit may not be a true laser or the training is lacking.
(See Notes 3 and 4.)

Electrical Stimulation

Medical uses of electricity date back to the experiments of Benjamin Franklin, where electrical shock was found to cause involuntary twitch and contraction of muscles. While Benjamin Franklin discovered the many benefits and uses of electricity, including treatment of gallstones and limb paralysis, I doubt he had veterinary applications in mind in the mid-1700s.

The application of safe electrical current over muscles, nerves, skin, and wounds is a modality commonly used in physical therapy for human beings and now animals. Both direct (galvanic) current and alternating (faradic) current are given with modulations in wavelength, frequency, and voltage levels. Electrical stimulation is effective in the treatment of pain, muscle spasm, muscle weakness and atrophy, swelling and inflammation. For the purposes of physical therapy in animals, two basic types will be explained: TENS and FES.

Transcutaneous electrical nerve stimulation, or TENS, is used in the treatment of pain. Specifically, it is used to modulate pain. It stimulates the sensory nerves via electrodes that are placed along neural pathways or on acupressure points and trigger points. TENS works on the gate theory of pain control, whereby the stimulation blocks pain messages from reaching the brain, at the level of the spinal cord.

Functional electrical stimulation, or FES, is also known as neuromuscular electrical stimulation (NMES) and as electrical muscle stimulation (EMS). This type of electrical stimulation is used to increase muscle bulk, strength, tone, and re-education of motor contractions. It is used in the following instances: after cruciate ligament surgery or hip surgery where muscle atrophy and weakness are present; for a tight and contracted rotator cuff injury; cases of sciatic nerve injury with "dropped paw"; after spinal surgery to retrain muscles, and more.

The FES and NMES types use alternating current and stimulate muscles through flat surface electrodes, placed strategically by the therapist. They work specifically on innervated muscles, where the nerve connection is intact. EMS uses direct current, which is needed when a muscle is denervated. All of these work by electrically stimulating a motor point, which is the place where the nerve enters a muscle, or by direct muscle fiber activation. Electrical current is generated by a stimulator that travels through wires (called "leads") to electrode pads or probes. When stimulation reaches the motor point, it causes depolarization and subsequent activation of the muscle fibers to contract. You will actually see and feel the pet's muscles twitch, vibrate, or contract. It does not hurt, if administered properly, and animals tolerate it quite well. The electrodes must make sufficient contact with the skin to overcome its resistance, so fur or hair must be shaved prior to treatment. It isn't necessary to shave completely down to the skin, and short-haired animals can often be treated with electrical stimulation without shaving at all. The therapist can help with shaving the region needed for treatment or can provide a diagram for the groomer or vet tech to follow. The electrodes will be prepared and placed, secured to the skin and hair by straps or self-adhesion. Tape should not be used to secure the electrodes. Some electrodes are a black carbon type, and need to have gel applied to their surface. Others, which are preferable in my opinion, are self-adhesive and more flexible; they can be trimmed to a specific size, and are highly conductive. In both cases, consistent surface contact must be made and the gel evenly applied or adhesive backing be smooth, without cracks, or burns and hot spots will occur. The stimulation unit will then be adjusted by the therapist for the correct parameters needed. These parameters are waveform, amplitude, pulse width or duration, pulse rate or frequency, polarity (positive, negative), and ramp (time from zero current to strongest amplitude). There are also time parameters: on/off time and treatment time. Adjustments in stimulation "on" and "off" will correspond to the way a muscle normally contracts and relaxes. A typical setting is five seconds on, followed by eight seconds off. Treatment time can be from five to fifteen minutes. The unit will be turned on and adjusted very slowly, along with soothing verbal assurances to the animal, until the desired effect is achieved. The therapist will look and feel for muscle responses that are effective and well tolerated by the patient.

Electrical stimulation should not be used over areas of skin irritation, in animals with pacemakers, over infected areas, over tumors, over the trunk or abdominal region during pregnancy, or over blood clots, and should be used with caution in animals with seizure disorders.

One more type of electrical stimulation, iontophoresis, used commonly in human physical therapy, is starting to make its way into the veterinary field. This uses ions, electrically charged particles, to deliver medication across and through the skin. Direct current, using an active electrode filled with the desired medication, and a passive electrode placed nearby to complete the circuit, are attached to a phoresor unit. Polarity is key, with the opposites attract and likes repel principle used in the medication delivery. If the medication carries a predominately negative chemical charge, the therapist will use the negative electrode as the active electrode. The medication injected into this electrode will then become repelled and transmitted from the electrode pad, through the animal's skin, and absorbed into the underlying tissue. The medication will be prescribed by your veterinarian, in liquid form, and given to you to bring to each therapy visit. Iontophoresis is normally used with anti-inflammatory medication such as dexamethasone, pain relievers such as lidocaine, and joint-relieving agents like hyaluronic acid. Mild redness over the area of skin where the active electrode was placed during treatment is normal, and can last twelve to twenty-four hours.

Massage

Massage has always been a cornerstone treatment for physical therapists. It is one of the first courses a PT student takes when beginning professional coursework. The benefits of massage to human beings with various medical conditions has been well received for decades and is now being utilized more in the animal world. Yes, animals "knead" it too! The benefits pets receive from massage are many of the same benefits that humans do, such as decreased tension, pain, and inflammation; increased blood flow and healing; decreased swelling; and reduced fibrous adhesions. And you can never underestimate those non-tangible benefits of the healing touch that calm, sooth, and allow the body to heal itself.

The technical definition of massage is "soft tissue manipulation or mobilization" and involves moving the hands along the skin and moving the underlying tissues, directed toward a specific purpose, aimed at achieving a physiological and psychological change. In animals, it is generally done in the direction of hair or coat, but sometimes done in the direction of the heart.

There are five basic types of massage:

1. *Effleurage or Stroking:* This technique utilizes gliding motions using the therapist's palm and fingers. It is excellent for removal of swelling and increased lymph drainage. It improves circulation and produces a flushing out effect. Bear in mind that the weather plays a role in affecting the soft tissues. When the barometric pressure in the atmosphere is low, tissues tend to swell and become more tender. If your dog is arthritic, you may notice its symptoms seem worse on low barometer/ humid/damp days and better in dry or high barometric conditions. Massage can be used to combat the uncontrollable effects that the weather has on your dog. Therapists may be likely to use this type of massage technique for swollen, tender tissues.

2. *Petrissage:* This technique involves kneading, compression, and skin rolling using thumbs and fingers. It is best for soft tissue tension (commonly referred to as spasm or guarding), and nodules, etc. They form from repeated strain, injury, and microtrauma that cause muscle tightening. This tightening is the body's natural reaction to trauma, shifting from a relaxed to a protective mode.

If the tightened, protective mode continues for very long without relief, the muscle becomes overused and fatigued, and changes start to occur within the cells. Within skeletal muscle cells are protein molecules called actin and myosin. These are small filaments that are organized into units of muscle tissue called sarcomeres. In turn, they are arranged in series, overlapping each other, like a ratchet system. This is the mechanics behind muscle contraction. Upon injury with muscle guarding and spasm, the cells simply start to run out of energy, so they secrete excess protein and the sarcomeres tighten up on each other (think of those brightly colored little woven Chinese torture tubes you may have played with as a kid, where you insert your fingers on each end and as you pull apart the tube gets tighter and tighter). Mild to moderate tightening that can be relieved by applying gentle pressure is called "guarding." Harder tightening that tends to feel very hard and worsens with pressure is spasm. Guarding and spasm usually occur in an entire muscle belly and it can't relax without intervention. Small concentrated formations of tightness can occur within the muscle called "nodules" or knots. They can also be called "trigger" or stress points.

So, how to cure this problem? From a physiological standpoint you want to flush out the excess protein and elongate the sarcomeres. This can be accomplished by the use of physical modalities like heat or cold, ultrasound or laser, massage, stretching, and muscle length rebalancing. The muscle also needs rest. This is why it sometimes seems to take longer to heal a muscle injury than a broken bone! A bone can fairly readily be rested through casts and splints, but muscles can be flexed even with restricted movement from a cast or sling, via isometric contractions. In severe instances medication may be needed such as muscle relaxers, injections, or dry needling techniques.

3. *Tapotement*: This technique uses tapping, cupping, vibration, and shaking using sides of hands, fist, or heel of hand. It can include gentle squeezing and wringing. These techniques are used on more dense, thicker areas of muscle tissue such as the thigh and hip or buttock area. It is generally used to relax very tense areas and sometimes used over the ribcage in respiratory conditions.

4. *Cross Friction or Transverse Friction*: Used for adhesions or scarring. It uses the thumbs and index fingers perpendicularly across the direction of the fibers. It can be uncomfortable for your pet but usually yields good, fast results.

5. *Connective Tissue and Myofascial Release*: Many therapists consider this to be of a type of manual technique but I have chosen to include it in the massage section due to its soothing and healing effects on the particular soft tissue called fascia. Fascia is webbing or a woven network of deep connective tissue that surrounds virtually every structure in the body: organs, ligaments, blood vessels, nerves, etc. This fascia is an organ of sorts that is dynamic, and transmits and adapts to mechanical stresses. When it becomes tightened or irritated through trauma, stress, or disease, adhesions form in the fascia and result in pain. An experienced physical therapist will be able to determine through careful palpation, observation, and movement if your pet has a fascial

restriction and might benefit from manual release. The technique is performed with the therapist's hands in various manners, such as applying gentle pressure and stretch over the skin and fur, rolling and gliding the skin between fingers, and arm-over-arm cross-hand tension with light force. This will be a comfortable technique for your pet and when performed properly, yields quick results. (See Note 5.)

6. *Lymphatic Drainage*: Here is an advanced technique requiring special medical training. This is used to help relieve a particular type of limb swelling or lymphedema seen in conditions such as cancer. It involves an initial clearing technique at the lymph node site, followed by a unique pumping type of massage that starts at the distal end of the limb near the paw and works up toward the proximal or the part closest to the body, and the heart.

Who should do animal massage? Veterinarians, physical therapists, massage therapists, and other health professionals who have received massage training and instructions. Giving a proper massage requires study of animal anatomy, medical background, and where/how to apply the various therapeutic techniques and maneuvers. It also takes practice. As a pet owner, your health care professional or vet can show you some basics for your particular pet's needs and issues. Please understand that without prior basic instruction, massaging your pet can do more harm than good. I have often been asked to give mini lessons to groups on animal massage but have declined for this very reason. In addition, you can never fool animals and they really know when the hands touching them are trained. The animal should be relaxed and trusting for the healing touch to have the best effect and they will not fully relax if they sense you are not prepared. I cannot stress enough that an animal always knows trained hands. A trained practitioner should pay close attention and listen for the feedback animals give.

One of my first and most poignant examples of this was with a camel! Yes, a very tall twenty-eight-year-old Bactrian, two-humped camel named Princess. I had never worked with a camel before (and I think most physical therapists could say the same thing), when I was asked to assist a Reiki practitioner who had been providing services to Princess for pain relief of arthritis and Lyme disease. Two sets of hands were needed to soften and release tension in her hard-to-reach scapular muscles of the shoulder blade and left elbow. I admit to feeling a bit intimidated when approaching Princess for the first time, unsure of how she would react to a new person laying hands on her, etc. The Reiki practitioner told me that Princess would know right away if I had good intentions, by my hearing my speech, smelling my breath, and observing my mannerisms. I was instructed to speak naturally to her as she began to lower her head down to my face, to give me my first inspection. As that great head came toward me with gorgeous eyes and long lashes, I stood very still and told her how pleased I was to meet her and that I would do my best to help relieve some of her aches. She seemed to sense that I was a friend and relaxed patiently as I began to palpate and feel for the location of her sore, guarded trapezius muscles. Although I had never massaged a camel before, I certainly knew how to massage animals and lovely Princess seemed to know this right away and she accepted me immediately. I also learned her habits and how to sense when she needed to shift and move (which becomes pretty important if you want your feet to remain intact!), or if she started to get irritated by outside distractions such as a goose standing atop her foot or a llama getting too close, all wanting attention. Princess wanted her massage and Reiki team all to herself!

When should massage be avoided? During fever, shock, active bacterial or viral infections, distemper, neuralgia, fungal skin conditions, open wounds, or conditions where there is acute and severe inflammation (need to wait a day or two for the inflammation to be less acute).

Ultrasound

The word "ultrasound" probably conjures images of pregnant bellies and images on a screen. The type of ultrasound used by a physical therapist is therapeutic, and of a different frequency than that used for testing. Ultrasound is inaudible, acoustic, mechanical vibrations of high frequency that produce thermal and non-thermal physiological effects. Therapeutic ultrasound frequencies range from 0.7 to 3.0 MHz, where diagnostic ultrasound frequencies range up to 10 MHz. Ultrasound waves are produced by means of a piezoelectric crystal. The crystal is located in the sound head, attached to a handle that is held in the therapist's hand. It is, essentially, a transducer, in which alternating electrical current causes the crystal to vibrate and emit ultrasound waves.

The therapist can choose from two forms of ultrasound: continuous and pulsed. The decision on which method to use is based on the desired tissue response. The continuous mode is a form of deep heat, which elevates tissue temperature, and increases blood flow and nerve conduction speed. It also increases extensibility of collagen fibers, resulting in greater range of motion. The pulsed mode minimizes heating effects to reduce scar tissue and areas of swelling. Once the mode has been selected, the therapist then selects an intensity, which is measured in watts per centimeter squared. Low intensity ultrasound is used for acute injuries, mid-range for sub-acute, and higher intensity for chronic stages. The next setting the therapist chooses is depth of penetration, measured in MHz: the higher the MHz frequency, the more superficial body structures absorb ultrasound. In other words, higher frequencies do not penetrate as deeply. So, if your dog has a strain in a muscle that is closer to the skin's surface, the therapist will choose a higher frequency (3 MHz) that penetrates only one to two cm. On the other hand, if the dog has arthritis in the stifle or hip joint and penetration is needed at a deeper level such as three to five cm, a lower frequency (1 MHz) will be selected. The time duration of treatment with ultrasound is relatively short: three to ten minutes.

Ultrasound cannot be used over metal implants or internal metal sutures, buckshot, etc. Metal objects near the field of treatment should also be removed as it concentrates the sonic energy and can cause burns.

Topical medications such as hydrocortisone cream or dexamethasone can be applied to the skin with ultrasound, called phonophoresis, as a medication delivery method. Pulsed ultrasound is used in this method, to drive the medication into the skin and to the underlying soft tissues in order to reduce pain and inflammation.

There are a few challenges in using ultrasound in animal treatment as opposed to human treatment. The first is that the hair or fur must be shaved very close to the skin. The sound head must maintain good contact with the skin so that acoustic waves are absorbed evenly. In addition, a water-based coupling agent is required to transmit the sound waves into the animal, or they will simply deflect off the body, due to natural resistance in the skin. Many pet owners are not fond of having their animal closely shaved and the pet doesn't always like the feel of cold, wet gel. Also, the sound head must be kept moving, especially if the continuous mode is chosen. If the animal moves suddenly and the sound head breaks contact, a hot spot of energy may occur, causing a sharp sensation. Despite these negatives, ultrasound is a very effective modality for use in the physical therapy treatment of animals.

Heat versus Cold

"Which is better to use: heat or cold?" This is a question that a physical therapist hears countless times during her career. The answer is...well, it depends! The key is to understand the physiological effects of each application.

Cold application, also referred to as cryotherapy, constricts blood vessels thereby reducing inflammation, controlling bleeding, and reducing sensation. It slows cellular metabolism and decreases conduction along the sensory nerves. It reduces redness and warmth, which occur when the capillaries release histamine upon injury. Cryotherapy is best used in the immediate hours after an injury or post-surgery, known as the acute phase. Examples of cryotherapy are: ice packs, cold whirlpools, ice massage, or water-cooled cold compression pumps. The benefits are seen with immediate pain relief, reduction of swelling, and ease of movement. Cold treatments are applied for approximately ten minutes, several times per day, for up to forty-eight hours.

There are instances where cold treatments should not be used:

1. In animals that are very sensitive to the cold weather
2. Cases of nerve damage or compromised circulation
3. Over open wounds
4. For animals that are very young or very old

As swelling decreases and intense pain subsides, the patient can transition to the use of heat. Heat applications elevate the temperature of tissues and dilate blood vessels, which increases blood flow to the treatment areas. This is beneficial in the sub-acute and chronic phases of healing, when inflammation is no longer present or minimal. Heat causes improved extensibility of soft tissue such as muscles and tendons, along with connective tissue, or fascia. This makes it very easy to apply stretching and other exercises that help reduce stiffness. It is quite common for a therapist to instruct you to apply heat treatments at home, prior to having your dog exercise. Heat is applied through various commercial hot packs, heating pads, warm wraps, or sacks. They can be filled with gel, silicon, ground cornhusks, and buckwheat. These are heated by hot water immersion or microwave ovens. Electrical heating pads can also be used with constant supervision, on the lowest setting available. Some heat wraps have iron filings or small discs that produce heat by contact with the body and an oxidation reaction occurs, producing heat for several hours. Most heating packs are applied for ten to twenty minutes, twice per day. Padding is required to prevent burns, adjusted to the amount and length of the animal's coat. They should feel warm but never hot. You will be advised to place your hand between the pack and your pet's skin to test the temperature after a minute or two of applying the pack.

All of these examples of heat application are considered to be superficial and penetrate up to one to two centimeter (one-half to three-quarters of an inch) depth below the skin surface. If an animal requires a deeper level of heat, the therapist will utilize ultrasound or laser therapy.

Heat should never be used in the following instances:

1. During acute inflammation (generally the first forty-eight hours)
2. During states of hemorrhage or the presence of blood clots
3. Over tumors or malignant tissue
4. Over open wounds
5. Over areas of decreased sensation

In general terms, heat is usually safe to use after forty-eight hours from an injury. When in doubt, your veterinarian or therapist will guide you accordingly.

Extracorporeal Shock-Wave Therapy (ESWT)

ESWT, like ultrasound, uses sound waves to treat medical conditions. That is where the similarities end. It is used primarily to break down areas of hard calcification or scar tissue. ESWT produces high-energy, focused sound waves that travel through the skin. When these waves meet tissue of different, harder densities, the energy contained in the waves is released. This produces a mechanical effect that helps to break down and obliterate solid tissues like calcium deposits, small bone spurs, etc. This result does not occur with just one treatment, but over a course of several sessions. ESWT is administered through a clear plastic cone and does not require use of gel and shaving like ultrasounds do. The ESWT generator is positioned and stays still in one position as it directs the acoustic pulses at specific tissues. Some generators are equipped with ultrasound positioning systems. The delivery of ESWT is through energy units of millijoules per millimeters (mj/mm2) and number of pulses delivered (200–250 pulses).

Most clinicians tend to use ESWT for chronic or long-term presence of tendonitis where calcium deposits have formed. Because ESWT is a focused stimulant and uses a high-pressure acoustic wave, it can cause some irritation after treatment so it is not likely to be used for acute or early-stage conditions. I have seen it used often in the equine industry and have applied it on rabbits, dogs, and goats with some success. Animals tolerate it fairly well, although some are initially startled by the clicking or tapping sound the generator makes. In terms of pain, the treatment, as perceived by human beings, is slightly uncomfortable to painless. My experience is that animals are more put off by the sound than the sensation. Although some ESWT treatments use high doses to achieve a similar-to-surgery effect and require anesthesia, the sessions provided by a physical therapist do not use sedation and are not as intense.

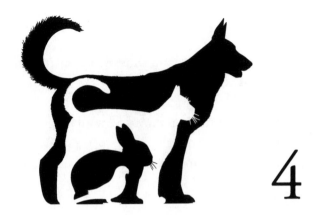

4

Types of Therapeutic Exercise and Manual Techniques

Range of Motion

Every joint in the animal's body is designed for movement and has a normal amount of scope that it moves through, which is referred to as range of motion, or ROM, of a joint. There are documented values, by degrees, that are considered to be the optimal standards for each of the joints. All animals function best when their ROM is within these normal values. However, when illness, surgery, or injury take place, the animal is less active and over time, its joints become stiff and lose normal ROM. Conversely, joints may become unstable, dislocated, and too loose due to trauma or disease.

During the physical therapy evaluation, the joints are examined and range of motion is measured with a goniometer. The joints determined to be tight and not in the normal value range will benefit from specific ROM exercises. The following is a general description of ways in which joints bend.

The shoulder joint moves in three planes of movement and five directions.

1. Extension: the arm moves forward and up toward the head
2. Flexion: the arm moves in a backward direction toward the tail
3. Abduction: the arm moves away from the body, out to the side
4. Adduction: the arm moves close to and across the body
5. Rotation: the shoulder turns inward and outward to achieve Internal rotation and External rotation

The elbow is a hinge joint and moves in only one plane, with two directions.

1. Flexion: bending
2. Extension: straightening

The carpus or wrist joint moves in three directions.

1. Flexion: bending down with the paw tucked in toward the body
2. Extension: bending up and back as if the paw is in a wave position
3. Deviation: the paw moves from side to side
   a. Radial Deviation: toward the body
   b. Ulnar Deviation: away from the body

The hip moves similarly to the shoulder:

1. Flexion: the thigh moves forward and toward the stomach and ribs (knee to chest)
2. Extension: where the thigh moves in a backward direction toward the rump
3. Abduction: the thigh moves away from the body
4. Adduction: the thigh crosses under the body, as in scissoring
5. Rotation: turning inward and outward for Internal rotation and External rotation

The stifle or knee is a hinge joint like the elbow:

1. Flexion: bending of the knee
2. Extension: straightening of the knee

The hock or ankle joint bends in several directions, but the two main ones are as follows:

1. Cranial Flexion: toes up direction, where the paw bends toward the head
2. Plantar Flexion: toes pointed direction, where the paw points away from the body, toward the tail

Here are the normative ROM values for each of these joints:

- Shoulder Extension: 165 degrees
- Shoulder Flexion: 50 degrees
- Shoulder Abduction: 45 degrees
- Shoulder Adduction: 40 degrees

- Elbow Flexion: 35 degrees
- Elbow Extension; 165 degrees
- Carpus Flexion: 32 degrees
- Carpus Extension: 196 degrees
- Hip Flexion: 50 degrees
- Hip Extension: 162 degrees
- Stifle Flexion: 42 degrees
- Stifle Extension: 162 degrees
- Hock Cranial Flexion: 40 degrees
- Hock Plantar Flexion: 165 degrees

Knowing the normal ROM values can be helpful in giving you some perspective on your pet's status by comparing the actual degrees measured by your therapist and veterinarian. Bear in mind that there may be some variations with certain breeds. For example, within the Jack Russell Terriers there are two body types: the rough- and broken-coat Terriers have longer, straighter limbs and stand with the stifles and elbows fully extended. Stifle and elbow extension for them is likely to be 170 to 180 degrees. However, the smooth-coated Jacks tend to have shorter bowed limbs and joints that do not fully extend. Normal stifle extension for the smooth coat is probably closer to 158 to 160 degrees. Your therapist can help determine more fully how the normative ROM values compare to your particular pet's breed.

Abnormal range of motion is characterized by being either too tight—hypomobile—or too loose—hypermobile. In cases of hypermobility, the joint needs to be rested and restricted from excessive motion by use of splints or wraps. With hypo-mobility, joints need to be exercised in order to gain flexibility and movement. Range of motion exercises will be employed, where the joints and surrounding muscles are moved through their available ranges. This movement may be passive, active, or active-assisted.

Passive range of motion exercises are performed by external force (e.g., a therapist's hands or mechanical device) and without any participation by the animal. This is used when the animal patient is unable to move joints on its own or if self-movement is painful or detrimental. Passive ROM is also used to help relax a patient who is tense or anxious.

Proper technique is very important when passive ROM is performed. The therapist must cradle and support the limb to avoid jarring or twisting stress on joints. Hands must be placed on both sides of the joint, with the end closest to the body held still and the end farthest away being moved. The ROM exercise should be smooth, slow, and steady, with the animal patient relaxed and comfortable. You may be wondering: "How does an animal stay still during passive ROM exercise?" The answer is simply that they inherently know and recognize trained hands. If they feel and sense your skill, they naturally surrender to your care. This does not mean that only a therapist or veterinarian can perform passive ROM exercises. A pet owner who is willing to learn can be taught to perform basic ROM at home, but he or she should be carefully instructed and supervised several times. Written instructions should be given or video of the exercise recorded for the owner. Passive ROM exercises are usually performed for five to ten repetitions, two to three times per day. Any pet owner who is uncomfortable doing this type of joint motion should be open and honest about it and never forced to perform ROM on his or her pet. It is better to spend the time and money having a professional provide this service than to have it done incorrectly and risk injury to the animal. There is no shame in admitting to feeling queasy about this. The only shame is to neglect having passive ROM exercises done when they are needed.

The other two types of ROM are active-assisted and active. Active-assisted ROM occurs when the therapist guides the animal's joint motion and the patient's muscles assist to a partial degree. Unless an animal is paralyzed or extremely weak, it typically contracts its muscles and moves with the therapist during the exercise. Active ROM is achieved by full muscle contraction by the animal. Placing a treat or toy in a certain position can stimulate the animal to move its limb on its own, through ranges of motion. Also, walking in sand or water, over rails or through a tunnel can achieve active movement through a joint's range of motion.

All ROM exercises are performed up to the limit of a joint's available range, whether done by passive, active-assisted, or active method. Additional pressure applied to the end of this range is called stretching.

Stretching

Stretching is used along with ROM exercises to increase flexibility of soft tissues: muscles, tendons, and connective fascia tissue. It is indicated when range of motion is limited by shortened soft tissues to help them elongate. Soft tissues become adaptively shortened in response to immobilization in casts or splints, illnesses requiring cage rest, during healing from injury, and sometimes because of excessive use in sports. Scar tissue and adhesions also form between the tissues and tie them down, preventing normal gliding and reducing motion. Neurological conditions can also cause tightness and shortening. When severe shortening occurs with very limited range of motion, it is termed a contracture. A theoretical example of this is a dog having hip surgery without good post-operative care who adapts to walking on three limbs, holding the operated-on rear limb tucked underneath the body. After a few weeks of this tucked-under carriage, the dog will develop flexion contractures at the hip and stifle.

Muscles, tendons, and fascia connective tissues are designed in overlapping, web-like units of fiber. Muscles have additional internal structures called "spindles" that monitor speed and the degree of stretch, and react accordingly. When these tissues are exposed to external stretching forces, their elastic component becomes elongated. With safe, repeated stretching, the over-lapping, web-like fibers actually rearrange and stay in their new position, resulting in tissue elongation.

Stretching is different from ROM exercise in that it takes tissues beyond their available range. It is most often performed statically (static stretching), with the limb held still. A limb or body part is placed in a position where the tissues are stretched taut to their greatest length, then held for several seconds. Initially the hold period is five to ten seconds and can be increased to as much as thirty seconds. It is repeated three to five times. Static stretching must be performed carefully and slowly to avoid injury. The limb must be held fully supported and properly aligned so that the animal stays relaxed during the stretch and doesn't resist. It is typical to allow a fifteen- to thirty-second rest period between stretching.

Stretching can also be performed ballistically (ballistic stretching) or with bouncing. This is a tricky maneuver, with some risk of tissue micro-tear, but is very effective for hard and dense contractures with a lot of deep scar tissue.

Stretching should only be done by a therapist or veterinarian initially, so that a safe determination can be made as to when the animal is ready in its recovery cycle. After it is clear that the animal can tolerate stretching, stay relaxed, and receive benefit from it, the pet owner can be instructed to follow-through at home. The results of stretching will be seen in successive sessions, with slow and steady gains in soft tissue length. The therapist can use a goniometer to measure the achieved increases in mobility and document the animal's progress in its medical chart.

Joint Mobilization and Manipulation

These techniques are used along with ROM and stretching exercises to increase joint mobility. They are indicated when range of motion is limited by stiff, tight joints and help to regain joint play. In healthy joints, there are imperceptible micro movements of gliding, rolling, and shifting that occur between the curved surfaces at the ends of bones that form the joint. These movements are referred to as "play." In addition, the joint surfaces are curved in concave and convex shapes, allowing them to conform to each other. A strong knowledge of anatomy is required as the direction of pressure applied in mobilization or manipulation depends on whether the joint is concave on convex or convex on concave. For example, the shoulder being a ball-and-socket joint has a convex-on-concave arrangement between the humerus head (the ball) and the shoulder blade socket. The stifle or knee joint has the opposite design, as the tibia is curved inward to line up with the round bulb-shaped ends of the femur bone in the thigh, making it a concave-on-convex joint. Joint mobilization and manipulation must be performed only by professionals (veterinarians, physical therapists, chiropractors) trained in these highly skilled maneuvers. Courses that teach mobilization and manipulation are beyond entry-level and found in postgraduate curriculums.

In order to increase motion in a tight joint, passive movements are performed within the patient's available range. These are oscillatory motions made with light to moderate pressure, using the therapist's hands, and are called "mobilizations." When performed repeatedly, and followed by passive range of motion and stretching exercises, increases in joint mobility are achieved.

Mobilizations are scored in Grades 1 through 5. During the technique, the therapist will move the joint through its available play, applying pressure and various degrees of rhythmical bouncing and springing and gliding motions. Grades 1 and 2 take place within the first half of the range. Grade 1 uses small amplitude and fast and light movements whereas Grade 2 uses larger, slower movements. Grades 3 and 4 are similar, but applied in the second half of the range. The best way to visualize this range is by imagining a rubber band stretched halfway to being taut (Grades 1 and 2), then stretched all the way to fully taut (Grades 3 and 4). When the rubber band is at its limit and about to break, it is symbolic of Grade 5. Manipulation is a Grade 5 maneuver, where the joint play is at its very end, or its breaking point.

Manipulations refer to techniques that are high velocity thrusts, which are performed at the limits of the patient's available range of joint play and beyond. Manipulations achieve increased joint mobility by this force, quickly and dramatically. However, these techniques require a great deal of training and skill and carry risk if not applied properly. Manipulations generally provide faster results than mobilizations, but the improvement can be short-lived. Manipulations often need to be repeated at various intervals to hold the improved alignment and mobility.

I admit to having a personal bias in favor of joint mobilization. The results take a bit longer, but the gradual nature of gaining play in the joints seems to affect their ability to retain the increased movement. No one knows if this is a pure physiological effect or more neurological in nature, where the joint learns to adapt to its new state. In addition, mobilizations are comfortable for the animal and make it easier to stay relaxed during treatment. I do use manipulation fairly often, but in combination with mobilization and stretching techniques. There are purist clinicians who perform only manipulation to achieve results, but most physical therapists employ a philosophy that a combination of techniques is the safest and most effective strategy for joint dysfunction.

There are contraindications for mobilization and manipulation to be aware of: These should never be applied in cases of joint fusion, any undiagnosed lesion or tumor, acute inflammation or infection of joints, spinal cord injury, or joint instability (such as Wobbler syndrome).

Traction

Traction devices are used to relieve pressure on pinched nerves in the spinal cord and reduce symptoms of degenerative arthritic joints in human physical therapy. In animals, traction is performed manually, without the use of mechanical devices. It is applied to all portions of the spine to relieve pressure. In order to achieve this effect, one part of the spine is stretched and elongated, while the adjoining section is stabilized to provide counter-traction. For the cervical spine (neck), manual traction is applied by the therapist's hands while the pet is sitting or lying on its side. The animal's head and neck are gently lifted by holding the pet under its chin and jaw while the therapist holds its shoulders and ribcage still. For pets that have dental or jaw problems, the therapist handhold is changed to the sub-occipital area, located just under the back of the skull. The head and neck are lifted slowly, with enough tension to cause separation between the spinal joints. This position is held for five to fifteen seconds, then gently released while maintaining full support of the head. It is repeated several times over the next few minutes. When done properly, this procedure is very comfortable for animals and extremely effective. Cervical traction should only be performed by your therapist or veterinarian.

Thoracic and lumbar (low back) traction can be taught to the pet owner to perform at home. It is applied with the animal lying on its side, stomach, or back, depending on the therapist's judgment of what is the most effective position for that pet. Basically, an elongation pull is applied to the pelvis, while the ribcage is stabilized, creating counter-traction. If the animal is large, such as a Mastiff, I often ask for assistance in the technique: having the pet owner hold the dog's shoulder blades and ribcage, while I apply traction force from the pelvis.

Positional traction can also be applied using a rolled towel or foam roll placed strategically under the pet's spine while they rest. Balls and Physio-rolls can be used to elongate the spine while the pet lies in position, stretched over on its side or stomach. Finally, traction can be applied gravity-assisted by holding the pet's head up, securing it under the arms and ribcage and allowing the lower body to hang, semi-supported against the owner's lap or body. All of these techniques must be provided initially by the therapist until it is clear that the animal can tolerate traction and is benefiting from it. Then you will receive instructions on how to perform traction at home and be asked to demonstrate it to ensure safety for your precious pet.

Contraindications for traction include the presence of bone disease or fragility of bone, active infections, spinal tumors, joint dislocations, or unstable joints in the spine.

Strengthening

Gone are the days when I would simply place a weight on one of my human patients and instruct them to lift three sets of ten reps! Strengthening exercises were a lot easier to administer with people. Animal patients present unique challenges that require creativity and ingenuity in overcoming language and attention barriers during the performance of strength exercise.

The extra effort is well rewarded in the results attained with strengthening exercises. Animals can achieve increased active range of motion, improved use of their limbs and core, correction of lameness, increased bulk and tone of muscles, better ability to function in daily life, and added benefits of injury prevention.

The basic types of strengthening are:

- Active: The animal moves its body part freely in space, on its own volition. The movements would be directed in a certain manner or direction to strengthen the desired muscle group.

- Active-Assisted: A therapist or per owner's hands would guide or help the animal during the exercise movements.
- Active-Resisted: An outside force is applied during movement to provide a barrier or resistance, thereby challenging the muscle to perform to a desired level (sub-maximal, maximal). The resistive force can be applied through position, manually or mechanically. Positional resistance is provided by gravity force. Manual resistance is provided by the therapist's hands or body weight. Mechanical resistance is provided by weights, sandbags, stretchy bands, or tubing.
- Open Chain: This is a general term used to describe a strengthening exercise performed where the limb moves freely through space, without the paw or foot attached to the ground.
- Closed Chain: These exercises are performed with the paw or foot making contact with a fixed point such as the ground or a platform. This causes strengthening throughout the kinetic chain, or system of overlap and interconnection of muscles and joints.
- Eccentric: This refers to exercises that invoke a specific type of lengthening muscle contraction. This usually involves a downhill or step-down activity where gravity is the defining force and muscle groups act to slow the body momentum.
- Functional: This involves whole body movements that mimic daily life activity. They will be discussed in detail in the following section.
- Plyometric: These are bouncing, jumping, vibratory, and landing exercises that are of a high velocity, rapid-reaction nature.

Principles used in the design and selection of strengthening exercises for animals are very similar to that of humans. The basics are intensity, frequency, and duration. Intensity refers to the amount of resistance or force the muscle must overcome to complete a movement. If using sandbags or Velcro-cuffed or strapped-on weights, the following guide is helpful in determining safe amounts of resistance:

- 10–20 pound dog or other animal: ½-pound weight
- 20–30 pound dog or other animal: 1-pound weight
- 40–60 pound dog or other animal: 1½-pound weight
- Over 60 pounds: 2-pound weight

In addition to the amount of poundage used, the location of weight attachment on the limb must be considered. Think of the limb as a lever arm: you know from life experience that holding a heavy weight with your arm extended out in front of your body is much harder than keeping it close to the body. Placing a one-pound weight on a dog's carpus (wrist) or hock (ankle) joint is much heavier and harder to lift than if it were placed just above the elbow or stifle (knee). Gradually introduce the weight to allow your pet to become familiar and used to it.

Many clients ask me, "How should I progress the weights?" "Is the guide (above) simply the starting point from which to add more poundage?" Well, because dogs and most other animals cannot clearly communicate a pain or strain response and are programmed to perform to please, adding more pounds of weight can be dangerous. The safest approach in using resistance is to keep the amount of weight constant and change the location of its placement on the limb. Start by placing the weight in a proximal location, closer to the body, and as the animal improves, reposition it farther out on the limb, in a distal location. It gives the old saying "out on a limb" true meaning! This is especially important in a post-cranial cruciate ligament (CCL) repair surgery or femoral head osteotomy (FHO) where a therapist is concerned about torque and stress placed on a healing joint. In these cases, weights are always proximally placed above the surgery site. Also, combining the use of weight resistance with other activity such as walking, slow jogging, and playing in sand or water can increase the effective intensity.

Resistance tubing and bands such as Thera Bands can be used in addition to or in place of weights, looped around the limbs in corresponding locations as described above. Thera Band products are made of latex and come in various colors relating to thickness and tension. Here is a guide to the Thera Band colors from easiest to hardest:

Yellow: thin, light resistance
Red: medium resistance
Green: medium/heavy resistance
Blue: heavy resistance
Black: extra-heavy resistance
Silver: very thick, super-heavy resistance

I recommend using only the yellow, red, and green bands for strengthening in rehabilitation programs. Blue and occasionally black bands can be used with healthy, athletic performance animals for enhancement programs. These animals should be of medium-to-large stature with good joint integrity to safely exercise with blue or black bands and ideally should be cleared by a therapist or veterinarian prior to use. I do not recommend use of the silver bands in animal exercise at all.

In cases of animals that are very weak and unable to lift a weight, resistance is supplied by Mother Nature in the form of gravity. Active-assisted strengthening, where the therapist or pet owner uses her hands to guide the animal's movements in space is a form of strengthening in itself. When the animal gains more strength the movements can progress from assisted to active where the pet moves on its own. This is a bit tricky but can be facilitated through visual aids such as toys or treats, using voice commands, and tactile or touching techniques over the muscles such as tapping, tickling, brushing, vibrating, or stroking to elicit a movement. For small animals that have delicate builds such as house rabbits and domestic cats, I do not use weights at all for strengthening, but employ functional exercises instead.

Each exercise can be performed for about five repetitions with a ten-second rest, and then repeated for several sets. Five sets of five reps generally works well.

Frequency and duration of strength programs varies according to stages of recovery, type of medical condition, etc. If an animal is very weak and debilitated, several short exercise sessions, five to ten minutes each, per day will be needed. Animals that have progressed beyond the acute stage and are ready for use of resistance and weights generally tolerate a frequency of one long session, fifteen to thirty minutes, every other day. If pain or irritation after exercise is present for one to four hours, there is no need for alarm. After another session or two, the pet will accommodate and should no longer appear to have symptoms. Pain lasting longer than a few hours and into the next day is a sign of too much intensity or duration. Lighter exercises, fewer repetitions, and shorter length of exercise time will solve the problem. Varying the routine and changing the order of exercise can also help prevent boredom or repetitive injury.

Strengthening exercise precautions include:

1. If your pet is on anti-inflammatory medication, these exercises are safe as long as they do not cause stress to joints and muscles. Using lighter resistance and placing weights above painful joints will reduce the possibility of strain.

2. Strengthening exercises should not be performed while your pet is taking pain medication/pain killers, as these medications mask pain and you will not be able to judge if the activities are causing injury until it is too late. Consult with your veterinarian: if the pain medications are given on an as-needed basis, you may be able to simply withhold giving the meds until an hour or two after the exercise session has ended.

3. Ideally, all strengthening exercise programs should be designed by a physical therapist or rehab-trained veterinarian for maximum safety and effectiveness. They can be carried out at home in many cases after the initial instructions are given. It is best to have a recheck in two to three weeks to monitor progress and tolerance to exercise. Exercises that require specialized manual facilitation techniques must be performed by a qualified therapist.

Here are a dozen examples of strengthening exercises:

1. Knee-to-chest or leg-lifting movements with the pet lying on its side, with a weight strapped around the limb, used to strengthen the hip and thigh muscles.

2. Tie Thera Bands or tubing around the wrists or ankles, or above the elbows or knees and have the animal take steps

forward, sideways, or back. This can be used to target various limb and trunk musculature such as the hocks.

3. Attach Thera Bands or tubing to a chest harness or loop around one or both thighs and provide resistance, while the animal walks. This helps strengthen the chest, hip, and thigh muscles.

4. Pulling a sled or cart attached to a harness. The harnesses must be well padded, and the animal able to maintain good position of the head and neck. Weights can be placed in the cart, or bags of dog food or sand used to provide resistance. Carts, especially with larger wheel diameters, are easier than flat sleds or small-wheeled carts.

5. Backpacks loaded with weights or sandbags can be used while a dog is walking, for strengthening. However, weights must be evenly distributed and kept light. This should not be used for dogs or animals with spine problems. Your therapist or veterinarian should be consulted before initiating backpack exercise.

6. Use of a sling or strap to raise the good or stronger limb off the ground and forcing the animal to use its weaker side can be a good form of strengthening, for short periods only. A coin or plastic cap can also be taped to the bottom of the paw on the good side, to achieve a similar effect.

7. Hills and slopes are great forms of resistance for strengthening: up the hill improves the short hip muscles in the hind limb and the rear triceps muscles in the front limbs. Going down hills, especially having the animal pause on a downward incline is a good eccentric exercise to work on thigh control and front limb, chest, and shoulder

strength. Initially, guide your pet in zigzag curves, while descending, for easier tolerance.

8. Walking through tunnels or under tables, like squatting while moving, strengthens the quadriceps muscles in the front thigh on the rear limbs.

9. Walking through tall grass (take precautions for ticks), in sand or on dry, powdery snow strengthens the hip and shoulder flexor muscles, those that contract to lift and progress a limb. It also improves coordination and endurance for your pet, as it navigates through varying types of terrain.

10. Hiding a favorite treat or toy in the sand or dirt and having your dog dig for it is a good form of strengthening for the shoulder and shoulder blade muscles.

11. Controlled ball play or other activity such as walking in figure-eight or circular patterns, using a leash or enclosed area, provides general strength and conditioning.

12. Provide gentle, slow hand resistance on your pet's shoulders and hips while it is standing still, challenging it to maintain and isometrically hold its balance. Change sides or direction after about five seconds. This is a fun game that strengthens the trunk and mid-body muscles. (See Note 6.)

Functional Exercises

If you have ever heard a physical therapist or fitness instructor refer to functional exercises and wondered what it meant, you will discover it here. Not only are these helpful to human beings in physical rehabilitation or sports enhancement programs, they are also used in pet recovery and fitness.

So, what are they? For an exercise to be considered functional, it utilizes the full body, using dynamic movement. It is an activity that replicates or mimics something that a person or animal normally performs in his or her daily life. It is performed without weight or machines, relying on the body's weight and gravity for resistance. In human physical rehabilitation after an injury or surgery, this type of exercise can also be referred to as "closed kinetic chain," and examples include squats, lunges, step-ups, etc. These exercises do not replace stretching, isolated muscle-specific strengthening, or cardiovascular conditioning. They are one component of a total exercise program, needed not only in rehabilitation but also in maintenance of overall fitness levels. Think of functional exercises as those that link the entire body in a manner that carries over into everyday activities.

Why are they important? They are safe, relatively simple, and do not require expensive, elaborate equipment. They are efficient not only in terms of time, but also in improving performance by working multiple muscle groups together, optimally as cohesive units. They prepare your pet for daily life movements, reducing potential injuries, strains, etc.

Below are various examples of functional strengthening exercises, but first a word of advice and caution. It is good to be educated and aware of all possible types of exercises but even the most basic can potentially be harmful depending on a particular animal's medical condition, age, breed, etc. For example, some of these might not be appropriate for a developing puppy, a geriatric pet with cardiac issues, a dog with spinal disc conditions, instabilities such as Wobbler's, and so on. Ultimately, a program should be designed and guided by your vet (especially if he or she has received rehabilitation training)

or an animal-trained licensed physical therap
sulted your veterinarian. These professionals w
the activities and give you initial guidelines o1
and other parameters so you can implement the program wiuı
your pet at home safely, with a favorable outcome.

Step-Ups: Use a raised platform such as a pallet, hard plastic
or wood box, oversized thick book, or similar object that is
approximately 15 to 20 percent of the height of the distance
measured from the ground up to your pet's withers. Have the
pet start off by placing one front paw up onto the platform,
then the other, and then paws back to the ground. During this
exercise, the rear legs stay on the ground. Example: up one,
up two, down one, down two. Although it will appear to be
strengthening the front limbs, it actually builds the thoracic
and lumbar spine extensors and hip/upper thigh musculature.
This can be advanced to having the pet completely climb up
on the platform with all fours, and then back down, repeated
several times.

Sit to Stand: Best done from a tight corner with the pet's hind
end backed into the corner. Repeat five to ten times. If you do
not have a good corner to use, place the pet's stronger side next
to/against a wall and have it stand from there. You may find
that some instructions tell you to place the weaker, surgical
side next to the wall, but I have found that placing the strong
side next to the wall forces the pet to shift weight away from
the wall and on to the weaker side, achieving a better result.

Dancing: You can hold your pet's front paws, but I prefer
holding the pet's upper arms, just below the shoulders for better
control. Have the pet hold the dance position in a standing
still (or static) position. Then sway from side to side or in the
dynamic position. Progress the exercise by having your pet

take dance steps with you going forward, to the left, to the right, and backward. Backward (or retro) dance walking is the hardest. Dancing can also be performed in a pool, with chest-high water level.

Wheelbarrowing: This involves standing behind your pet, holding up the hind limbs, and having the pet bear weight on its front limbs. You can gently guide your pet forward to take a few steps with its front paws. Be careful and check with the vet first if there is elbow dysplasia or spinal conditions.

Weight Shifting: While your pet is standing on a piece of foam or thick carpet, gently pick up a front paw; hold for a few seconds, and then place it back down. Repeat with the other front paw. After that, lift a back paw, followed by the other. Progress the exercise by simultaneously lifting an opposite front/back paw at the same time, called "contralateral" (left front paw with right back paw). Follow this by the right front paw with the left rear paw. Final progression is lifting both right paws at the same time, then both of the left paws, called "ipsilateral." You can also use a foam mat or pad four- to eight-feet long, one-quarter to one-half-inch thick, then thicker as the legs get stronger, to encourage higher hip flexion by the pet actively raising up its paws, also called "high stepping." Have the pet walk back and forth on it, turning around at the end. You can also try using a toy or treat to have the animal take some steps backward on the foam.

High stepping: This can also be performed over a ladder placed horizontally on the ground, or logs spaced a few feet apart, or low hurdles.

Toys for Functional Play: One of the best types of this play is playing tug of war. Using a braided rope toy, the game encourages the dog or pet to crouch down, bending knees and elbows, and moving sideways (lateral) and backward. Use caution if there are any dental or neck issues. If your pet likes to play with balls, you can quickly roll a small ball sideways between your palms to encourage the pet to lunge from side to side in response, following the ball.

Rolling: Assist your pet to roll from side to side, initially by placing your hands on its shoulders and hips. Progress this by using a toy or treat and moving it from side to side over the pet's head, encouraging it to roll and follow the toy. You can also hold the toy or treat over the tummy area and have your pet reach for it, simulating a partial curl-up. These exercises will work the abdominal core region of the body.

Timed Up and Go (TUG): Use a stopwatch (you may have this function on your cell phone) to time your dog, starting from a sitting position at a distance of eight to ten feet away. Ask the dog to come to you and measure the speed at which it stands up and comes to you across the room. This is a basic measure of mobility skills and is helpful for older arthritic pets that show slower movements in getting up to stand. Make it a fun game for them, gradually getting faster. Currently there are no standards for this test in the animal world, so just start with your pet's initial time as your baseline and try to increase it 5 to 10 percent per week. In my experience, an older arthritic pet should be able to do this in seven to ten seconds.

Functional strengthening activities offer great variety for your pet to exercise efficiently and effectively from head to tail!

Swimming

Aquatic therapy using pools has become very popular in the animal rehabilitation field over the past eight to ten years. Water is a wonderful medium in which to exercise, offering warmth, buoyancy, and resistance. Many species and breeds of animals love being in the water (yes, even the occasional cat) and find great enjoyment from swimming and exercising in a pool. In addition to pools, animal aquatic exercise can take place in whirlpools, bathtubs, lakes, ponds, streams, and underwater treadmills (see Chapter 5). The benefits of water exercise and swimming include:

1. The hydrostatic pressure of water helps support balance and weak limbs so that an animal can move without falling.
2. Buoyancy, or the upward thrust of water, takes pressure off of sore painful joints affected by arthritis or healing from fracture.
3. Cohesion, or the binding force of water molecules adhering to each other, provides resistance for strengthening. When the body moves through water, force is required to separate the molecules. Water is a relaxing and supportive medium in which to move and strengthen weakened muscles, especially if multiple parts of the animal's body have been injured or affected by a medical condition.
4. Water has a high specific heat and temperature conductivity so that it is able to heat or cool the body core rapidly.

The following are also precautions and contraindications associated with aquatic therapy and swimming:

1. Your veterinarian should always be consulted prior to starting any swim or aquatic program, whether medical and rehabilitative or recreational related.

2. If surgery has taken place prior, all incisions should be closed, sealed, and dry prior to any water applications, in order to prevent infection or the possible spread of bacteria, etc. These incisions may not be fully healed internally yet, but as long as they are closed well and considered to be sealed by a veterinarian, therapist, or pool manager, it should be safe to swim.

3. Some species, such as cats and individual canine breeds, may be frightened of the water and could become agitated, thrash about, and potentially harm themselves. These animals should be identified and not subjected to swimming or aquatic therapy.

4. Pool activity should be supervised at all times.

5. Diarrhea, bowel and bladder incontinence, bleeding, vascular disease, and heart or lung conditions are contraindications.

6. Any medical or health conditions that may be affected by heat and humidity should be contraindications to aquatic therapy.

7. Laryngeal paralysis with tie-back surgery is absolutely contraindicated for swimming. The larynx is the anatomical opening to the trachea (windpipe). When it is impaired by paralysis and tie-back surgery is performed, animals are not permitted to swim as the larynx would not be able to close if the head submerged under water and drowning could occur.

Conditions also exist where swimming might not be contraindicated, but is not the best choice for a patient. Sometimes therapists deal with situations where well-meaning pet owners or guardians have their own ideas and decide to go in another direction away from the therapist's recommendation. For example, I had a fascinating case involving a fostered Jack Russell terrier named Markus, who displayed weak and contracted hind limbs along with abnormal motor tone and spasticity. Markus's hind legs were so disabled that he literally walked only on his front limbs, with his rear legs bent and tucked under his body and not even touching the ground! It was a strange sight and puzzling to his veterinarian and entire care team. After numerous tests including muscle biopsy, blood work, and radiographs, the diagnosis remained a mystery. A working diagnosis of dystonia (a neurological muscle contraction disorder) was the basis for developing ongoing treatment with medication prescribed by the veterinarian and physical therapy that I provided consisting of relaxation and stretching of the hind limbs and weight-bearing exercises. It wasn't very long before Markus began walking on all four limbs with partial weight bearing on the rear limbs. He further improved in using his limbs in a reciprocal left-right pattern, instead of bunny hopping, and was able to jump onto a chair.

Then rather abruptly, Markus's care was transferred by his foster guardian, resulting in a change of venue for his veterinary care and physical therapy. The guardian decided that water therapy and swimming would be more beneficial. I was not consulted, but if I had been given the opportunity to give my opinion, I would have said that swimming would probably not help Markus because the water buoyancy could not provide the needed weight-bearing and stretching activity he needed. Markus received swimming therapy for about six months and did not improve. He was eventually transferred back to the care of the veterinarian who referred him to me and we resumed physical therapy. Markus also found a new forever home. The moral of the story is this: Not every condition can be defini-tively diagnosed, but every clinical decision must be based on principle and have sound reasoning behind it. I love swimming for animals, but I include it in a treatment plan only when there is a justification for it and not simply because it sounds like a good thing to do or to see if it will help.

In terms of the need-to-know specifics of pool swimming and aquatic exercise, I have gone to my source, Angelina Ruggiero, manager of a canine swim facility in New Jersey, who has many years of experience in this field. The following is an interview I conducted with Angelina, to find out the latest information and advice:

Author: "Angelina, how many years have you been involved with helping dogs swim?"

Angelina: "I have been swimming dogs for nine years. I started out as a customer when our veterinarian asked me to swim Stella, my Chocolate Lab, because she needed to lose weight. A few months later, she was diagnosed with hip dysplasia and the vet continued to highly recommend that she swim. What started out as recreation for my dog turned out to be not only my new career, but I realized my passion was in helping dogs! Swimming is not only for dogs, but horses and other animals too."

Author: "Can you give readers some guidelines to look for when choosing a good swim facility for their pet such as pool size, water temperature, etc.?"

Angelina: "There are many variables: size and energy level of the dog; the purpose of swimming and whether it is for recreation or necessity; whether the facility offers both private sessions and group swim. The water temperature should be between 75 to 80 degrees in the winter months. Owners should consult with their veterinarian before starting a swim program if their dog has any medical conditions to ensure they are safe."

Author: "How should pools like this be cleaned and maintained?"

Angelina: "Chemical levels should be measured and balanced daily. Pool skimmers must be cleaned several times a day and the pool should be vacuumed and backwashed as needed."

Author: "What questions can pet owners ask about beforehand to ensure the experience is safe and secure?"

Angelina: "Is there a staff member present at all times? Are aggressive dogs given private swims? Are life vests required for the dogs' safety? How is the facility maintained and cleaned between swims? What is the policy with dogs that have bowel or bladder incontinence? Some facilities charge a fee to cover draining, cleaning, and refilling the pool if a dog has an accident. This can run up to $400 at some facilities. Other facilities do not swim incontinent dogs at all. Are staff members familiar with basic anatomy and medical conditions of animals, and are they willing to collaborate with the veterinarian and physical therapist?"

Author: "What types of life preservers and other safety equipment are used?"

Angelina: "All dogs are required to wear life vests. I prefer Outward Hound and Ruff Wear. Since humans do not swim in the pool that I work in with their dogs, leads are required for all new dogs and dogs that are compromised. Leads are attached to the life vest (not to the dog's collar) to provide for a safe and controlled swim. By the way, muzzles should not be used when swimming a dog. Owners also need to keep in mind that not all dogs can swim, so safety equipment is extremely important."

Author: "What ancillary facilities should be present in a full-service aquatic swimming facility?"

Angelina: "Bathing stations should be provided if the pool is chlorinated, along with a place to dry your dog (especially in the cold winter months). There should be a ramp to allow the dog to gradually walk into the pool, with treads and side walls."

Author: "Does each animal have its own individual swim time or can it be handled in groups?"

Angelina: "It depends on the situation: for example, aggressive dogs must swim as a 'private' with their own individual swim time slot. It is very important to be honest with the facility staff about your dog's behavior; group swims are acceptable for recreation after the dogs personalities have been assessed and they are paired/scheduled accordingly."

Author: "Can you describe how a typical swim program is designed? What can you expect on the first visit? How does the program advance as the dog shows improvement, etc.?"

Angelina: "It depends on the size and shape of the pool. Laps can be linear, circular, and even diagonal. Our particular pool is circular and very large, originally designed to handle horses. So, one lap in our pool is equivalent to six or seven laps in a small pool or three to five laps in a medium-sized pool. The first visit we usually allow more time and start with a total of ten minutes of swimming, one large lap at a time. Sometimes the first visit is overwhelming for the dog so I feel it should be a private session. I ask clients to watch their dogs after the visit to see how they tolerate it. Some dogs just love to swim and will overdo it initially, their excitement being fueled by adrenaline and they won't display pain. So it is very important to start with a smaller amount of swimming, erring on the side of caution, especially with the first visit or two. Afterward, you can expect a dog to show some fatigue for a few hours, but they should not be exhausted for a whole day. The second swim is longer, adding five minutes, and gradually working up to thirty minutes.

"We also look for special parts of the swim that are challenging. For example, a dog that has had cruciate surgery usually has trouble making turns in the pool initially. We assist them and use balls or toys and verbal cues to help."

Author: "I've heard some therapists suggest placing a foam roll or noodle in the dog's mouth to help guide them to make turns or swim in a curve or circle, to strengthen the spinal muscles that help control lateral movement."

Angelina: "Yes, but any special foam rolls or other devices would normally be used on the advice or input given by the physical therapist. We swim dogs but we do not try to be physical therapists and we always collaborate with the dog's therapist and veterinarian."

Author: "Please share a noteworthy case you have had in which swimming played a dramatic role in a dog's recovery or illness."

Angelina: "Well, for me the most touching cases are those dogs that come in with neurological problems like degenerative myelopathy, usually Shepherds, Corgis, and Labs. One case I'll never forget is a dog named Snickers, a ten-year-old dog with neurological issues who was full of life but could no longer play ball or Frisbee and couldn't take long walks due to limb dragging and knuckling. On land, he would need braces or a cart but in the pool he could do everything. I remember when he learned to swim for the first time, it gave this dog such delight! By the next month, Snickers was able to jump in the water and catch his Frisbee again. He got so excited that he now had something he could do and it brought joy back into his life. We often see neurologically impaired dogs come in the first time looking so sad and depressed until you show them they can swim and play in the pool. It opens up a whole new world for them. They wait every week to come back and do it again!"

Author: "Are those tears I see in your eyes?"

Angelina: "Yes, I can't help it. There is just no better feeling than helping a dog like Snickers to swim!"

Author: "Thank you for your compassion and skill in helping thousands of dogs swim!"

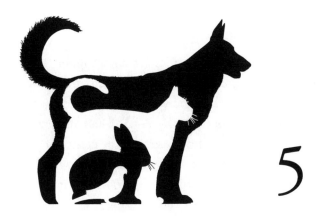

5

Use of Equipment in Treatment

Underwater Treadmills

Other than sharing the physical medium of water, underwater treadmill walking offers a very different form of exercise from swimming. Underwater treadmills are enclosed, self-contained units that allow a patient to walk partially submerged in water. The units have controls that alter the treadmill speed, depth, and temperature of water. Resistance from the water can be increased by adjusting the treadmill to a higher speed and by adding air jets. The ability to make all of these adjustments allows a therapist to systematically control how the animal exercises and keep records of progress.

Unlike swimming, underwater treadmill exercise is weight bearing, which is a closed kinetic chain type of strengthening activity. The amount of weight bearing varies by the depth of water. When a dog or other animal is immersed in greater depths of water, the weight bearing becomes reduced due to buoyancy. For animals with balance and weight-bearing problems, therapists will start with higher levels of water and gradually reduce the level as the patient improves. The animal can stand in the water and practice bearing weight and balancing on its limbs. A good starting level of water is below the withers and just above the center of gravity (mid-chest level). At this level, which is also hip level, the patient will nearly float but still be able to bear some weight, about 25 percent of that if on land. When the water is lowered to just above the knee, the patient will bear about 65 percent of that if on land. When the water is further lowered to just above the ankle, weight bearing is about 85 to 90 percent of that if on land.

In addition to weight bearing, underwater treadmills allow the therapist to focus on strengthening a particular body area by varying the depth of water. To target special body areas, a child's arm floats can be attached to the thigh, elbow, or shoulder. This causes that part to float and the pet must use its muscles to push it back down under the water. To strengthen the thigh or arm muscles, the water should be below the knees and elbows. To strengthen the lower arm and hind leg muscles, the water should be just up to or slightly below the wrist and ankle joints.

Please note that the physical therapist should get wet too. Although not required, I feel the best results are obtained when the therapist dons her thigh-high waders and joins the animal in the tank to provide reassurance and guide it through the learning curve of walking on moving treads. A floatation vest may also be added for safety. At no time should the therapist leave a patient unattended in the unit. (See Note 7.)

Land Treadmills

Regular treadmills, also called "land treadmills," are used with animals that have a higher level of functioning and are able to comfortably bear full weight on their limbs. Therapists find benefit in use of these treadmills for progressive training and control of performance. Inclines can be set to mimic walking up hills. Speed can be varied to allow interval training and endurance building. A specific pace and duration of the workout can be easily set, measured, and documented (and you know we therapists love this!) and reproduced. The land treadmill also offers the ability to exercise indoors, free from wind, rain, ice, snow, and other poor weather conditions.

If you are a runner or speed walker, you have probably noticed some differences in doing this outdoors on roads and streets compared to on a treadmill. At times, the land treadmill seems to produce lower heart and breathing rates, usually due to the loss of resistance from the elements (like wind). Also, the forward biomechanics of walking and running on land require the body to accelerate and decelerate, while propelling the body ahead. On a treadmill, there is no true propulsion as the belt of the treadmill cycles under the board and the body is essentially keeping up rather than pushing forward. So, there are some differences, but treadmill walking and running has merits and sufficient similarity to land walking.

For animals, treadmills should have low side guarding walls along the whole length of the unit as well as in the front. The walls should be high enough so the animal can't easily jump off but low enough that the therapist can have full physical access to guide and support the animal. A harness attached to a center pole or elevated arm support can be used to keep the pet centered. The treadmill should also have fine-tuning ability for speed control. Some also have advanced technology, embedded in the platform and belt, to detect and analyze lameness. These pressure-sensitive walkways, along with software, can pick up and record weight-bearing deficiencies that may not be easily observed during normal walking. As an evaluative tool, this special type of land treadmill can provide good information to assist in treatment planning as well as track and record improvements.

Land treadmills can be used for strengthening, general conditioning, endurance, weight loss, and weight control. Those manufactured for use with animals have special tread belts that will not scuff or irritate most paw pads. Along with walking, creative activities for advanced functioning or performance can be integrated into the program such as:

1. Reversing the animal's facing position on the belt to simulate backward walking (which can target the hamstring and hip muscles).
2. Front leg walking with only the front paws on the belt, while the hind limbs stay on the floor or elevated surface such as an inflated bubble, disc, or other type of platform. Speeds must be slowed for the animal to adapt to the challenge and maintain safe movement control. This type of exercise is used for a performance athlete and strengthens the chest and shoulder blade regions, as well as the trunk and core groups. For dogs or any animal that needs to perform turns, the therapist can hold a visual object or treat to one side, causing the animal to utilize its oblique abdominal muscles, needed for control during turns.

3. Rear limb stepping can be performed with the front paws placed on a surface as described above, and keeping the rear paws on the treadmill belt. The animal is facing the back of the treadmill. This adds a component of advanced strengthening for the upper back and sides, along with the triceps muscles along the rear of the upper forelimb.

As with all equipment exercise, a therapist or other qualified person should always be present while the animal is on the treadmill.

Before we leave this topic, a new type of indoor walking device is now on the market. It is a wheel, similar to what a hamster uses. A tread wheel is animal powered, fairly compact in size, requires no electricity, and offers an alternative to long treadmills. Animals can run at their own natural pace and there are optional brakes that allow for varying resistance to the wheel. The wheel comes in various sizes to accommodate toy through giant breeds.

Rails and Poles

Okay, you're probably thinking of torture devices and strip clubs at this point! Let me put an immediate stop to that by clarifying how rails and poles are used in physical therapy for animal agility and fine motor training, along with more traditional exercise in post-hip, stifle, and even spinal surgery. Balance, limb position sense, strengthening of the side flexor muscles in the spine, and coordination are all improved with use of vertical poles, so let's explore those first.

Weave poles can be fixed or flexible. They are usually mounted to a fixed bar or base and set approximately twenty-two inches apart. The fixed poles are easier at slower speeds and the flexible or slanted poles are challenging with brisk paces. Dogs are the primary species that use poles and for agility events, they are usually trained to enter the first pole to the left (dog's right shoulder is to the left of the first pole). The dog is trained to navigate alternately and smoothly around and between the poles, with a steady forward motion. A leash is used to guide them initially, along with verbal commands, and a clicker or treat.

If weave poles are not affordable or available, wooden stakes, PVC pipe poles, traffic cones, or bicycle racks can be substituted. Cones work well and can be used for weaving as well as figure-eight turns. The spacing of cones is farther than the typical twenty-two inches of the weave poles. For small dogs, I recommend placing cones three to four feet apart, medium-sized dogs five to six feet apart, and large breeds seven to eight feet apart. To make a greater challenge with tighter turns, gradually move the cones closer together.

Cavaletti rails, similar to those used with horses, are parallel raised pipes or poles, made of molded plastic or wood, spaced apart on the ground. They are used for small jumps or high-stepping motions to promote strength and coordination, and help lengthen an animal's stride. The height of the rails should not be above the animal's hock, or ankle joints. This allows sufficient height to challenge the muscles while avoiding strain to the spine or the risk of trips and falls. Initially, a leash should be used to guide the animals in stepping over each rail in a slow, controlled manner. As the animal gains proficiency, speed can be increased to trotting, but not to the point of hopping over each rung. The pattern should be a reciprocal left-right-left-right limb movement throughout the exercise. Use of rails is a great way to strengthen the flexor muscles of the front limbs—the biceps and deltoids—and of the hind limbs—the psoas and hamstrings. Ladders positioned flat on the ground can be substituted for Cavaletti rails. Floor ladders can also be specially made out of pressure-treated wood supports, with holes in which PVC pipes are threaded. Small hurdle sets are good simulators of Cavaletti rail–type movements and can be used well in therapy programs.

Physio-Rolls and Balls

Inflated, colorful Thera Balls (also called "Swiss balls") and Physio-Rolls offer wonderful variety to therapeutic exercise programs, both in therapy clinics and in the pet's home. The colors correspond to a variety of sizes, ranging from twenty-five to 105 centimeters. In selecting the right size for your pet, the top of the ball should be the same height as the shoulder blade or slightly below the withers. The optimal height allows support of the animal's spine and trunk, with some weight bearing on the paws and limbs. Occasionally, a larger size may be selected where the limbs do not extend to the floor, if total de-loading of the joints and elongation of the spine is desired. The other factor is shape: they can be round, egg-shaped, and peanut-shaped. Round shapes can be a bit more challenging for balance and the egg or peanut shapes are more user-friendly to the animal. There are also donut-shaped discs mounted on springy platforms and long cylindrical rolls made of foam or upholstery-covered fibers that are used during exercise programs.

Your therapist will select the size and shape of the ball or roll best suited to your pet and the type of exercise needed. Thera Balls and Physio-Rolls are used for stretching the hips and shoulders, weight shifting, traction and elongation of the spine, stabilization and strengthening of the core muscles, balance training, and helping your pet to bear weight gently on limbs that are weak or painful.

The amount of inflation is also adjusted to suit the stage of recovery or condition. Often a ball will be underinflated in the beginning sessions to make it easier to mount and get off of the ball, and provide less resistance. Balls and rolls can be inflated more, as the animal progresses. Weather has a factor in altering the inflation level, similar to your car tires; in winter, they might need air added and in summer, reduced. Most animals accept using the balls and rolls fairly well, especially if their owners are assisting or participating in the exercises. Occasionally a pet might be fearful and run from it and some might try to aggressively play and bite the ball. If a pet does not adjust to or tolerate it, a different form of exercise should be substituted.

Here are some examples of exercises done with use of the balls or rolls:

1. The pet is placed with chest and stomach over the ball, while it is rocked forward and back or side to side, helping it balance and learn to bear weight on its limbs.

2. The pet may be placed on top of the ball or roll, standing on all fours with the therapist or pet owner holding it securely under the chest and ribs, while it is gently bounced. This promotes the abdominals and core muscles to contract and stabilize the spine.

3. The pet can stand on the ground with its hind limbs, while the stomach and front limbs are placed on the ball or roll. This helps to strengthen the rear limbs and increase hind end awareness and weight bearing.

4. The pet is placed with its rear limbs and stomach over the ball, while its front limbs and paws remain on the floor. This provides some assisted, graded weight bearing on the front limbs and chest, helpful in shoulder stretching as well as strengthening of the elbows and carpus (wrist) joints.

5. Treats, clickers, toys, and praise are used to guide the pet to look up, down, or turn from side to side, as directed by the therapist in fine-tuning the exercise to target certain joints or muscle groups.

Balance and Rocker Boards

Rock and roll takes on a whole new meaning when applied to exercise instead of music! Rocker boards, wobble boards, Balance Bubbles, BOSU platforms, and others share a common goal in attainment of proprioception. Proprioception is conscious awareness and sense of the limb's position in space or on the ground or other surface. Structures called "sensory receptors" are present in joints and ligaments throughout the body that pick up signals from various types of stimuli as the body moves and encounters forces. The receptors help the body to respond in order to shift weight and balance. A body can be trained to better adapt to stimuli through exercises that are performed on moving, unstable surfaces. Therapists use devices such as a rocker board, with a low fulcrum point and a non-slip surface on which to place an animal and rock it from side to side, front to back, diagonally, or in a circular motion. Boards with higher fulcrum points are available for larger breeds and to advance small to mid-size breeds to a greater level of challenge. In addition to boards, inflatable bubble surfaces are also used to challenge balance and improve proprioception. The movements are done slowly and gently to help the pet gain awareness of the changes in position. The movements are never done in a rapid, spinning, or jerking motion. Some boards have raised sensory points on the platform surface to provide additional stimuli to the joint receptors. This will be done with constant hand contact on the pet for safety and calming measures, until they learn how to shift weight and balance safely. These boards come in various sizes to allow all four paws on at one time, and can have low walls or fencing around the perimeter. Other times, a smaller board will be used and only part of the body positioned on the platform, with the other half maintaining contact with the ground. This allows targeted proprioception workouts for a specific region such as the hocks (ankles) or carpus joints (wrists).

There are other uses for these boards and bubbles in addition to balance and proprioception, namely stretching, strengthening, and weight bearing. The back and forth rocking can be a good way to stretch the shoulder, hip, hock, or carpus without the animal even realizing it, which helps in pets that are anxious during hands-on techniques. This is considered an indirect approach, offering an alternative way to reach a goal. Focused strengthening of the hock muscles can be achieved through rocking forward and back while allowing the heel to drop down off the platform. Rocking also allows an alternate method of training a pet to bear weight on one particular part of the body or toward one side, through the shifting, swaying movement. These devices are versatile, portable, and relatively inexpensive, offering a form of exercise that can be reproduced at home as well as in the clinic.

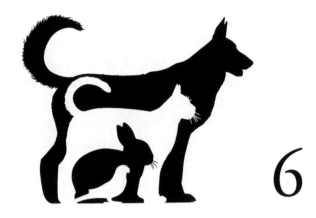

6

Rehabilitation of Orthopedic Conditions

Compensation and Symmetry

Harmony and balance: isn't that what everyone really desires? Your beloved animal companion gives you a measure of that every day. Animals also need it in a physical sense in the way they stand, walk, and function. Their bodies, like ours, are designed for symmetry, in order to maintain structural integrity of joints, bones, muscles, etc. What you see in the normal animal posture and gait is like a symphony orchestra where all parts blend into a harmonious sound. For pets, it results in a fluid, smooth pattern of standing and locomotion. In the orchestra, the best sound is achieved through coordinated effort. If one instrumental part is not attuned to the whole, a musical fault will be heard and, in order to go on with the show, other parts overcompensate in an attempt to restore relative harmony.

A similar scenario occurs in dogs and other animals when one area of the body is injured or missing (through amputation), and thereby challenged to maintain homeostasis. In order to have balance the body adapts an abnormal posture that compensates for the weakness by a redistribution of body weight. It is considered a strategy, or an adaptive coping technique. This can be observed with the pet standing still (static) and during movement (dynamic). During movement, there is a reorganization of the locomotive system, required in order for the pet to remain functional.

The basics behind maintaining homeostasis in balance is keeping the center of gravity (COG) over the base of support (BOS). The BOS is the stance position of feet/toes on the ground. The COG is the point in the body where mass is equally balanced or distributed in all directions. In a human, it is located just in front of the upper lumbar vertebrae. The canine COG is at mid-chest just behind the shoulder blades. It needs to be kept in optimal position over the base of support to maintain balance. Therefore, dogs always try to keep their COG just behind the front limbs. If the hind limbs are weak this pulls the COG backward. The dog will try to control it or compensate by shifting weight forward (cranially), toward the head, to try to return it to a normal place. The result is increased weight on the front limbs, beyond normal. (See Note 8.)

If this compensatory attempt goes on too long, potential problems can occur with overuse. There can be overdevelopment (hypertrophy) of the neck, shoulder, and scapular muscles; inflammation of the shoulder, elbow, and wrist joints; and a widened stance. Broadening of shoulders and positioning of front paws farther apart are attempts to widen the base of support during gait. As mentioned above, hind limb weakness is usually the source and occurs from ligament tears, hip dysplasia, spinal disc disease, etc. Sometimes widened front limbs are due to general obesity with large body mass. In pets with neurological impairments, the hind limbs will cross over or scissor, and the front limbs will widen to compensate.

A veterinarian or animal-trained physical therapist will make a systematic observation from the back, front, and side of the pet to analyze posture and assess gait as part of a total evaluation. The therapist's eyes and hands are her most important evaluation tools.

Therapists look to see if weight is evenly distributed on the hind limbs, if there is lowering of the hips and pelvis because of an injury and the muscles cannot support the hips, etc.

Normal weight distribution is 60 percent on the front limbs and 40 percent on the hind limbs (it can change to 70 percent/30 percent with hind limb weakness). For this reason, tripod amputees missing a front limb are more challenged than those with an absent hind limb. In fact, there is very little gait change in a hind limb amputee.

(See Note 9.)

The goal is to strengthen the weak areas and retrain the pet to shift weight back onto the affected area to avoid the compensation and restore symmetry. Here are some tips and exercises for hind limb strengthening:

> Strengthen the hip and thigh musculature through basic sit-to-stand exercises, using low calorie treats, a clicker, or a toy as a training aid for motivation. Repeat the movement five to eight times. Watch for symmetry, as the pet will tend to sit just on the stronger hip and rise toward that side. A good technique is to start from a tight corner, such as in your kitchen, so the dog can't cheat and use only the stronger side. Use a treat

and hand signals to walk the dog backwards into the corner first, and then ask it to sit, and then stand, etc. You can also have it sit with its stronger side toward a wall and when it stands, the wall will force it onto the weaker side.

An indirect way to force weight back toward the hind limbs is to alternately lift one front paw or limb and hold it up for a few seconds. Alternate between the left and right six times. You can progress to placing both of the front paws up on a low step or platform and have the pet hold the position for five to fifteen seconds. You may have to use a sling to support the hind section.

Ideally, you should have your vet or PT demonstrate these exercises before trying them at home. She should assess how the pet tolerates them and provide you with starting parameters as well as how to progress, etc.

Nothing beats the value of the controlled leash walk to increase hind limb strength. It should be done slowly at first, then increase to a comfortable pace, but always controlled. If the dog, for example, is limping, bobbing its head up and down with each footfall, or bunny hopping, you need to slow the pace until the proper gait is seen. Start for five minutes and gradually increase the distance and time, two to three times per day. Gradually add variations such a leash circles around a tree, making wide turns in a figure-eight pattern, varying the walking surface (grass or sand), and climbing up and down low grade slopes, hills, and inclines, to increase the strength.

Intervals can be added to increase endurance, consisting of short ten- to fifteen-second bouts of faster speed, every few minutes.

Many other exercises exist using sandbag weights, Thera Bands, carts, sleds, weave poles, Cavaletti rails, Physio-Rolls, rocker boards, treadmills, and more. They are best performed by an animal-trained physical therapist or a veterinarian trained in rehabilitation.

Hip Dysplasia

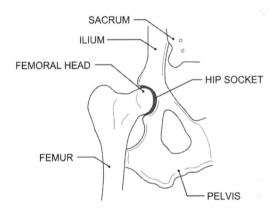

HIP JOINT

Figure 2

A common ailment found in dogs is canine hip dysplasia (CHD). The hip, consisting of a ball-and-socket joint formed by the head of the femur (ball) and the acetabulum of the pelvis (socket), is also called the coxofemoral joint. This joint is designed for movement and formed so that the shapes perfectly match each other, with the socket surrounding the ball. In human beings, who walk upright on two legs, with the hip in a neutral position or in a straight line to the body, the hip moves through a lesser degree of arc in walking compared to the dog. The canine walks on four limbs, with the hip in a bent or flexed position to the body, producing a greater arc of movement during gait. It is very important for the ball and socket to make good and even contact, in order to achieve the quality of movement needed for a dog to walk comfortably. (See Figure 2.)

In dysplasia, the acetabulum socket is shallow and abnormally developed. The femoral head, or ball, also becomes misshapen. The result is that the socket does not fully surround the ball and loses contact and coverage. This gets worse as the dog grows and the hip becomes loose and lax. In most cases, the hips appear normal at birth, but as the dog develops, the hips progressively lose contact and become unstable. The cause of dysplasia is through genetics and inheritance, seen mostly in large and giant breeds. Those breeds of dogs that have a rapid weight gain early in their development, such as German Shepherds, Labs, Rottweilers, and Saint Bernards, tend to show a high incidence of hip dysplasia.

Visible signs of hip dysplasia differ between puppies and dogs over one year of age. The puppy will tend to show lameness with running, jumping, and climbing. You will often see a bunny-hopping gait and may hear a popping or clicking sound. With an older dog, lameness will be seen more with normal walking. The gait will look short and choppy with less-than-normal movement in the strides made. The back end of the dog might even appear to waddle from side to side, as the pelvis is used to help bring the limbs forward and back, taking pressure off the hips. The rump and thigh muscles might also appear atrophied or shrunken. It is also very common for the range of motion to be markedly decreased when trying to pull the leg back, into extension.

Don't misunderstand: dysplasia is not the same thing as arthritis, but a dog over a year old that has dysplasia can form arthritis as a result. So, arthritis does not cause dysplasia, but dysplasia can cause arthritis! The long-term result of the laxity in the ball and socket is wear and tear on the hip with the formation of painful bone spurs, or osteophytes.

Canine hip dysplasia is diagnosed by veterinary examination and by radiograph (X-ray). Documentation and registry of this disease is important in the breeding industry. Breeders want to ensure that a dog is not at significant risk for transmitting dysplasia to its offspring. Two different testing methods are the OFA method from the Orthopedic Foundation for Animals, and the PennHip method, from the University of Pennsylvania Hip Improvement Program.

OFA maintains a large database of hip evaluations. Your local veterinarian takes the radiographs, following specific instructions, with the animal anesthetized and sends them away for an OFA evaluation and certification score. OFA radiologists review the radiographs for conformity, size, shape, and architecture of the hip joints. Three different OFA doctors will analyze the hips and assign a consensus score, relative to other dogs of the same breed and age. A normal hip is usually graded as excellent, good, or fair. Dogs with dysplasia are graded as borderline, mild, moderate, and severe. OFA evaluations are usually done with dogs over twenty-four months of age. They are not recommended for females during times of heat,

GREAT TO KNOW
"Canine hip dysplasia was first described in 1937 by Dr. G. B. Schnelle. Originally thought to be a rare condition, it is now recognized as the most common orthopedic disease in dogs."
—Penn Hip

pregnancy, or nursing, due to increased ligament laxity during these times of hormonal imbalances.

The PennHip method requires veterinarians to take a special training course to be certified to perform the test. Radiographs are taken of dogs as young as sixteen weeks, and utilize a distraction and compression view. Using weights and an external device, the hips are pulled away (distraction) or pushed in (compression) to determine the amount of laxity in the joint. The distance that the femoral head (ball) is pulled away is quantified using a distraction index (DI). This measures the amount of laxity in the hip and coverage of the ball by the socket. In addition, the higher the DI, the more susceptible the dog becomes to developing degenerative arthritis in the future.

Surgical options for hip dysplasia are the triple pelvic osteotomy (TPO), the total hip replacement (THR), and the femoral head osteotomy (FHO).

The triple pelvic osteotomy (TPO) is performed on young dogs, usually less than ten months of age, before any true damage has developed in the joints. During surgery, the pelvic bones are broken and the ball-and-socket joint is realigned to correct the alignment and position.

A total hip replacement (THR) is the best procedure for dogs that have painful degenerative joint arthritis. The surgery involves removal of the existing hip, replacing it with an artificial joint or endoprosthesis. The result is a functionally normal joint that is free from pain. The down side is that THR is very expensive and requires a longer recovery.

The femoral head osteotomy (FHO) requires a much more in-depth explanation. Femoral head osteotomy is the surgical excision (removal) of the ball and neck of the femur, at the hip joint. It is used in cases of advanced hip dysplasia where the hip joint has also become arthritic, in complex fractures, and for cases of avascular necrosis (lack of blood supply to the bone). A genetic condition called Legg-Calvé-Perthes, seen mostly in toy breeds, is an example of avascular necrosis.

When I get a new referral to see a canine patient post-FHO, two immediate questions come to mind: How long ago was the surgery? Are the dog parents realistic in their expectations of the outcome? From experience, I know that if the parents have waited a month or two (or longer) after the procedure to call me and/or are expecting their dog to walk as well or better than before the surgery, I am about to face some heat.

FHO is not the only option for these conditions, but it is probably the most commonly chosen. If I don't sound like a fan of FHO, you are right. But nobody, even the surgeon, is a fan of FHO. This is because it is a non-reversible salvage procedure and not a truly corrective one. Given the other options available, however, it is usually a very practical choice.

The other two options—TPO and THR—have high success rates, but involve longer recovery and are much higher in terms of cost.

The FHO becomes, if not the optimal treatment of choice, rather an economical solution with a shorter recovery period. It is performed more on smaller dogs of less than forty pounds, and not as highly recommended for large dogs. The key is to understand why it is being done and what to expect afterward. When the hip joint is damaged by one of the conditions described above and conservative measures have not been effective, the hip will continue to worsen without surgery. By worsen, I'm referring to degenerative changes such as arthritis, fragmentations, and bone spurs, which will become painful and debilitating for your dog.

When FHO is performed, the removal of the head and neck (the ball portion of the hip) allows a false joint to form in place of the normal ball and socket. From that point on, the hip is biomechanically altered and the leg becomes shortened. Even with physical therapy and rehab, there can be some recurring deviations and lameness in gait with less weight borne on the leg than before the surgery. Many times I have heard a dog owner ask, "My dog seemed to walk just like this or better before, so why did I have this done?" My response is, "Your dog is now free from pain and secured from future crippling arthritis and degeneration." Although, with FHO, the return to full function is limited, the quality of life is enhanced, and the owner still has his or her retirement savings intact!

At this point you may be wondering how the dog can sit or walk after FHO without the firm contact of the femoral head in the socket. Initially the animal will redistribute its position to bear weight more on the front limbs and other hind limb. This can lead to overcompensation so it is essential that physical therapy be started very soon after surgery to help the formation of a false fibrous joint. This is facilitated through early range of motion and weight-bearing exercises. The empty space fills in with soft connective scar tissue to form a new "pseudo" joint, which forms according to stimulation and stresses put onto it (Wolff's Law) such as range of motion and weight-shifting activities. The veterinarian and physical therapist can show the dog owner how to do some home exercises, along with scheduled rehab sessions. This can start immediately after surgery or ten to fourteen days after surgery when the sutures are removed, depending on the surgeon's protocol. If you choose to wait two to three months after surgery to see how it goes before deciding whether to try PT, it will be too late to maximize the formation of the fibrous tissue.

Along with early physical therapy exercises, you can apply moist, warm heat packs to the hip to help bring blood flow into the region. Be sure to place a thin towel over the shaved area first, then the heat pack on top, to avoid burns. The temperature should be warm, not hot. Plan for a quiet homecoming after surgery, especially if there are other pets in the house. Place carpets or non-skid runners over tile or wood floors to avoid your dog slipping. Pillows can be placed in several locations on the floor where your dog normally likes to sit, to help it ease to and from the sitting position.

Avoid the use of stairs initially and use a leash with a collar or harness for the stairs when the vet tells you to resume. Contact your vet for adequate medication for pain and inflammation, to allow your dog to handle the early exercises needed to maximize the formation of the false joint. This new pseudo joint will not have the stability of a normal hip, so running, jumping, and hard playing may become somewhat limited. But you can expect your dog to resume walking with near to full weight borne on the limb, for fair to good distances, and to enjoy a comfortable high quality of life.

There are a few other types of surgery for dysplasia, such as darthroplasty (dorsal acetabular rim arthroplasty) in which bone graft is used to deepen the hip socket.

Non-surgical management and treatment of dysplasia includes weight management, physical therapy and rehabilitation, and various drugs and oral supplements. Weight loss can be highly effective, often as much as use of drugs. Lifestyle changes such as avoiding slippery floor surfaces, eliminating jumping, enjoying daily controlled leash walks, and using the right dog bed can make a huge difference. Physical therapy treatments for dysplasia often consist of heat modalities, laser, massage, range of motion with manual joint compressions, swimming, use of a Thera Ball or Physio-Roll, gentle stretching, balance, and strengthening exercises. Physical therapy can be used in dogs having hip dysplasia, whether or not they have had one of the surgical procedures mentioned above. After surgery, the rehabilitation consists of the same treatments just described, but under different guidelines or protocols furnished by the veterinary surgeon. The progression of activities and techniques is designed to safely allow the dog to heal from the surgery and recover as quickly as possible with optimal results.

Cranial Cruciate Ligament Tears

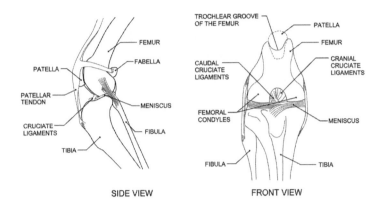

KNEE

Figure 3

Cranial cruciate ligament (CCL) tearing or rupture is one of the most common causes of hind limb lameness. The CCL, located in the knee (or stifle) joint provides stability by preventing forward slippage of the tibia, relative to the long thigh bone or the femur. The stifle is the most problematic joint of the body, particularly in dogs. It is a complex joint starting with the rounded shape at the end (like knobs) of the femur, the plateau of the tibia, the patella, meniscus, cruciate and collateral ligaments, tendons, and joint capsule. Because of this, some veterinarians and therapists embrace the concept of this joint being an organ. Here's how the structures work: the capsule protects the joint surfaces by being a mechanical barrier, providing blood supply and nutrition to the joint along with a lubricating fluid that gives viscosity for the joint to work. Ligaments provide support to the capsule and bind the joint together. The patella or knee cap rides in a smooth canal formed by a valley in the femur and provides a fulcrum for mechanical advantage to the quadriceps muscles when they contract. The menisci or shock absorbers are triangular wedge-shaped cartilage structures that transfer stress off the joint surfaces.

Now let's examine what happens and why things can go wrong with the stifle. The cranial cruciate ligament, correlating to the anterior cruciate ligament (ACL) in humans, confronts unique biomechanical forces in canine down-on-all-fours gait compared to upright two-legged human gait. The human ACL tears more acutely, mainly from trauma. The canine CCL tears from repeated movements; non-trauma related and acute tears are less common. This type of tear is usually a slow and gradual degradation followed by complete rupture. It is not only due to different forces on the stifle during canine gait but also from the shape and angle of the canine tibial plateau. In humans, the tibial plateau is essentially flat, and sits in a level transverse plane almost parallel to the ground. In dogs, the plateau is more sloping in shape and sits in a plane at an acute angle to the ground. Therefore, gravity affects the canine CCL differently with more shearing forces on it during walking on all fours than on the human ACL in upright gait.

Once the stability of the CCL becomes compromised, the stifle joint is lax (or loose) and the menisci can tear or degenerate because of repeated stress from the laxity. Patellar luxation in a medial or inward direction can also develop. With these problems, the first outward sign is non-weight-bearing (NWB) or partial weight-bearing (PWB) lameness in the affected limb. In turn, this causes increased weight on the other sound limbs, both front and back. Overuse syndrome can then occur, leading to inflammation, irritation, and crepitus (or sounding crunchy) during passive range of motion. Inflammation left untreated causes tissue damage by dilation of the blood vessels with release of histamine, activation of enzymes with release of free radicals that digest matrix and contribute to loss of cartilage and formation of unwanted scar tissue. This can progress into arthritis, or degenerative joint disease (DJD).

That is why dogs with a ruptured CCL have a 20 to 40 percent chance of tearing the other side! The incidence is also variable by obesity and by certain breeds that have some underlying genetic predisposition, but it is not just the large breeds. There is a correlation to body structure—straighter leg dogs of both large and small breeds have more chance of CCL tears than bowed. Breeds with straighter bones have more direct force on the ligament as opposed to breeds with more bowed bones like the bulldog, dachshund, or corgi. If the injured CCL goes untreated or is operated on but takes longer to recover, it's more likely that the other side may wear and tear beyond the 40 percent. If the injured side becomes arthritic, there is a 60 to 70 percent chance that the other side will tear within twelve to sixteen months.

The key to prevention of other side tears is in the *timing*: early diagnosis and surgical correction for complete tears, early post-op rehab, healthy diet, and ideal body weight. Otherwise, excessive weight shifted onto the sound leg will increase the possibility of that CCL tearing. If the tear is just partial and you see only intermittent lameness, surgery may not be needed, but PT with modalities such as laser, functional electrical stimulation, and massage can be of great benefit, along with other treatments advised by your therapist and veterinarian.

Diagnosis of CCL tears is made through observation, the performance of a drawer test, and with the help of radiographs

(X-rays) and MRI. The drawer test is performed using the hands and can be done by the therapist or veterinarian. The test becomes positive if the tibia slides too far forward, such as a drawer being pulled out from a chest. Grades of 0 to 5 are assigned, depending on the millimeters of excessive tibia movement demonstrated in the test. A partial tear might have a grade of only 1 or 2, whereas a full tear will likely score Grade 4 or 5.

CCL tears can be treated non-surgically and surgically. If the animal has a slight or partial CCL tear, non-surgical treatment is usually indicated. Initial rest, use of medications prescribed by your veterinarian, and physical therapy, along with braces or wraps can be used. Physical therapy is very beneficial in the use of laser to help facilitate healing at the tear site and reduce inflammation. Allow me to clarify: Laser will not help the torn ligament to reattach, but rather to strengthen and firmly bind the residual part still intact. It can also help form scar tissue over the torn portion, which helps give tensile strength to the joint. I have seen many dogs having partial tears with an initial positive drawer test of Grade 2, be reduced to a Grade 1 or even 0 after several sessions of laser. Laser, along with massage, range of motion, various strengthening exercises, and rigid adherence to restrictions in activity during the initial weeks after the tear, can yield favorable results. These same options are used in dogs with complete or full CCL tears that cannot undergo surgery for various reasons due to advanced age, seizure disorders, or stress-related conditions that pose a high risk for anesthesia.

It should be stressed that CCL tears that are not treated at all are at very high risk for developing degenerative arthritis. If surgery is not an option, you must seek other forms of treatment, such as physical therapy, braces, and animal stem cell transplants. Ask your veterinarian about physical therapy right away! Treatment should not be delayed.

Surgery for CCL tears is varied in the many approaches used. Your veterinarian will refer you to an orthopedic specialist, likely board certified, who can evaluate the tear and make recommendations for the best method based on the animal's size and breed, your budget, etc. There are two basic categories of CCL surgical procedures: intracapsular and extracapsular. There is a protective covering of tissue called a capsule that covers and surrounds joints, to seal and hold synovial fluid in. This helps maintain lubrication of these joints, along with stability. Intracapsular procedures (also called "4 in 1" or "over and under") are those that are done inside of the capsule, and require cutting it open, and then removal of the torn ligament; removal, repair, or release of the cartilage (meniscus); removal of bone fragments or spurs (osteophytes); reconstructing the ligament with grafts; and finally closing it. Intracapsular repair uses biological tissues or synthetic materials (e.g., Dacron and polyester) to internally reconstruct the ligament. Because the capsule is invaded, the surgery can cause inflammation associated with the graft and may pose a greater risk for infection and sepsis.

Extracapsular repairs include the big three: TPLO, TTA, and lateral suture technique. There are also the FHT and Flo procedures. Here is a general description of each:

TPLO: tibial plateau leveling osteotomy. This is a complex procedure that requires special training for an orthopedic veterinary surgeon. It is used often with larger breeds that are heavily built, such as Rottweilers. The TPLO works by changing the angle of the top of the tibia, called the tibial plateau.

This helps, through mechanics, to overcome the forward tibial thrust that occurs without an intact CCL. It provides functional stability of the stifle during weight bearing. The top, or plateau, of the tibia is normally sloped downward, to allow an optimal angle for the quadriceps muscle to function. The problem is that this also exposes the CCL to shearing forces, especially with larger, heavier breeds during times of heavy play, going up and down stairs, and so on. The TPLO levels the tibial plateau not by physically grinding it down, but by cutting a wedge section of the bone below the plateau and changing the angle by tipping it, realigning it, and fixating it so that the slope is more parallel in relation to the ground. There is a good degree of internal hardware used and the animal must usually stay in the hospital twenty-four to forty-eight hours before going home.

TTA: tibial tuberosity advancement. The tibial tuberosity is a bony projection on the front of the bone that serves as an attachment for the thigh (quadriceps) muscle. The advancement technique uses a special plate and spacer cage packed with bone graft, to move the tuberosity forward. This allows the quadriceps muscle to pull more at a parallel direction than at a sloped angle. This makes the muscle's new angle of pull tighter and acts more like a CCL ligament, in preventing forward thrust of the tibia.

FHT: fibular head transposition. This method surgically re-orients the top (head) of the outer bone of the leg (fibula) in a forward direction, where it is pinned in place. This allows the lateral collateral ligament, which attaches to this part of the tibia, to act as a mechanical barrier to prevent cranial drawer instability, similar to what the CCL would do. This is a fairly easy procedure and allows the limb to return to early function. Good range of motion for flexion and extension are obtained although the rotation of the joint is limited. There are some risks of clicking (crepitus) and fracture of the fibular head in about 12 percent of the cases.

Flo: modified retinacular technique. During this procedure an incision is made through the connective tissue (fascia) as well as through part of a muscle, and a suture wire is inserted and fixated to act as an artificial ligament. This uses an incision on the inside, or medial side of the stifle. The suture is attached to the patellar tendon (the knee cap tendon), along with the detached portion of the muscle and fascia. Other tissue nearby can be overlapped and sutured to cause increased tension, thereby providing support in the absence of the CCL. In my experience, the technique is used for smaller, lighter weight dogs as there is a risk for the suture to break with joint stiffness occurring. It also allows earlier rehabilitation as there is no ligament graft.

Lateral suture technique: performed on the outer (lateral) side of the stifle. This is a relatively quick procedure with good results. It uses a loop-type of leader line suture that attaches to the outside of the lower femur and at an angle down to the upper portion of the tibia. It provides good stability to the joint, in the absence of the CCL, but externally there is some bulk and can feel like a knot or extra piece of bone. As with all of the surgeries, it requires good attention to sterilization and occasionally results in failed procedures due to infection and sepsis. It seems to be a good alternative to more expensive procedures, in medium to large dogs, when economic concerns are relevant. The lateral suture is often used for feline patients with CCL tears. The feline cranial cruciate ligament is proportionally larger than a canine's and a cat's patella has a distinct tear drop shape. Many surgeons opt to use this method for cats, along with general surgical exploration and cleaning-up (debridement) of the stifle joint.

With a lack of historical data to determine the effects of long-term joint control, there is no clear-cut choice in surgery method and no obvious advantage of one particular technique over the others. You and your surgeon will have to consider many factors such as the animal's health, size, breed, lifestyle, age, along with financial resources and the surgeon's skill set.

Another topic that should be addressed is what to do about the meniscus. The meniscus or cartilage in the stifle is damaged about 50 percent of the time when the CCL ruptures. This is true of the inner or medial meniscus more than the outer or lateral one. Sometimes it needs to be removed or repaired at the same time of the CCL surgery. There is controversy about this as the meniscus serves as a spacer and shock absorber for the stifle joint and when removed, can cause wear and tear with eventual arthritis. Some surgeons will opt to keep the meniscus in place but release the back (caudal) portion of its attachment to the joint and capsule, to free it from strain and further damage. This last option may be the best of both worlds and should be discussed with your pet's surgeon.

After surgery, the physical therapy and rehabilitation typically begin upon removal of the stitches, at ten to fourteen days post-op. Your surgeon will give you written instructions on what to do during those first two weeks. It usually involves activity restriction, application of cold packs, medication instruction, and monitoring the surgical incision. Your pet may need to wear a cone collar to protect the incision and keep it dry. Any warmth, redness, or drainage at the incision should be immediately reported. During those first two weeks, the animal may or may not start to put weight down on the operated limb. You cannot let your pet run, jump, play with other dogs, or use the stairs. The surgeon will likely ask you to use a leash when taking your pet outdoors to do its "business." There should be no off-leash activity during that time before stitches are removed, unless it is indoors in a small, restricted area. If you have a large home, it is best to use a leash for indoor movement. Some surgeons will ask you to begin simple range of motion exercises during the first two weeks, but others may wait until the next phase of treatment.

During weeks two through six, increased weight bearing on the operated limb is allowed and encouraged. You can begin slow, short leash walks of five minutes, or up to one-quarter mile one to three times per day. The pet can start to use a few steps or stairs, only on leash. Running, jumping, playing, and interaction with other dogs should still be fully restricted during this time. Range of motion exercises should now be started. They involve bending (flexion) and straightening (extension) of the stifle joint and are best performed with the animal lying on its side. This is the point at which many pet owners decide whether to continue rehab on one's own or hire a physical therapist. Most are prompted to contact a physical therapist when the pet is not putting the limb down to bear weight; the leg muscles are weak and atrophied; or the stifle joint is stiff and the pet owner is squeamish about touching and moving the limb. These are perfectly sound reasons to seek professional help. I am not going to preach that using a physical therapist is essential for your pet's rehabilitation after CCL surgery. You can be successful following the surgeon's instructions in many cases. I will say, however, that using a professional therapist is optimal. You will likely get the fastest results with the best chance of avoiding injury or long-term complications such as arthritis. Also, bear in mind that you can use a physical therapist just to do the initial evaluation and instruct in a home exercise program, with some brief follow-up every two weeks or so. The usual scenario is to start physical therapy between the tenth and fourteenth day, with two sessions per week during the first two to three weeks, then reducing to once per week. Modalities such as cold or hot packs, electrical stimulation, laser, ultrasound, and massage will be applied, along with range of motion exercises and gentle stretching of the hamstring, quadriceps muscles, and the Achilles tendons. The therapist will use functional exercises and various techniques to facilitate having the pet bear the proper amount of weight on the limb. This will entail some weight-shifting and alternate limb-lifting exercises, placing the animal over a Physio-Roll, using treats and commands to encourage and teach the pet how to re-use the limb safely. You will be given instruction in how to follow through with exercises and activity between sessions. The therapist will continually monitor the incision healing and your pet's overall response to treatment progression. If any abnormal signs are seen, she will communicate immediately with you and your veterinarian. Sometimes things go wrong, such as post-op infection, but if caught early they can be quickly reversed. The value of a physical therapist in those situations is priceless.

After the sixth week and through week twelve, the animal should be at or near full weight bearing on the operated side. Leash walks can be increased to distances of fifteen to twenty minutes, or one-half to one mile, one to two times per day. Range of motion should be near normal values at this time. Normal bending or flexion is approximately 40 to 42 degrees, measured by the therapist using a goniometer. Straightening or extension is 160 to 170 degrees, depending on the breed. Your pet may be allowed on the stairs at this time, off leash, depending on the advice or your therapist or veterinarian. My criteria for allowing stair negotiation off leash is that the pet can perform this reciprocally (left-right-left-right) and not by bunny hopping with both hind limbs moving at the same time. Also, the pet must be able to bear at least partial weight on the operated limb and not simply carry it up. If the pet is not able to do a reciprocal gait with good weight bearing, then you should still use a leash for going up and down a staircase. Strengthening exercises will become more advanced at this point and involve resistance using hands, cuff weights, and exercise tubing. The Physio-Roll will be used in more creative ways, rather than simply placing the pet over it to bear weight: the pet may be placed on top of it and/or exercise with it in combination with foam rollers or balance bubbles. Inclines and hills will be added to increase hind limb muscle strength and bulk. Various circular, figure eight, and other movement patterns will be included in the treatment program. High-stepping over rails or low hurdles is helpful to increase the lifting of flexor muscles, while walking through a tunnel helps to strengthen the extensor groups. Limb lifts while the pet is standing will continue but become more challenging by rising more than just one at a time. For instance, the therapist might lift the front and hind limbs together on one side of the body (ipsilateral) or on opposite sides (contralateral).

At twelve to sixteen weeks the speed and distance of leash walks increases and can include trotting. Therapeutic activities might also include active play with tug toys and jumping across/over low obstacles.

By sixteen weeks, it is usually safe to allow full running and some jumping, provided the operated limb is fully sound, and on the approval of your veterinarian and therapist. Play with other dogs might be permitted if monitored carefully. There should be lifetime precautions imposed to prevent injury to the surgery site, including avoidance of running on wet grass or ice/snow-covered surfaces, jumping off of high levels, rough play, etc. Be mindful of keeping your pet's weight at a reasonable level and follow all advice regarding medications and supplements that your veterinarian recommends.

(See Notes 10 and 11)

Patellar Luxation

The patella is similar to the knee cap in human beings. When it slips out of place it is called "luxating patella." If this has ever happened to you or someone you know, you have probably noticed that it slips to the outside or lateral part of your knee and thigh. In animals, it tends to slip out of place in the other direction, or inner medial side of the knee (stifle). With humans, it occurs most often from trauma but in animals it is associated with developmental or congenital defects that are present from birth. Some animals are born with a smaller than normal patella and others with a shallow groove for the patella to sit in. In dogs and cats, the patella can luxate to the lateral side of the stifle, but this is seen only in cases of limb deformity. Patellar luxation is present quite often in toy and miniature breeds of dogs and in some cats as well. The patella serves as a fulcrum for enabling the quadriceps muscles of the thigh to contract efficiently. It is small, round in shape, and sits in a bony trochlear groove within the long femur of the thigh. There is a clinical grading system given to patellar luxation, depending on its severity.

Grade 1 is an intermittent off and on luxation, which can occur with simple handling of the limb and can be easily realigned manually or self-realigned by the animal. This is typically seen with a dog or cat shaking or kicking its hind limb in a back and upward direction, snapping it back into place. There is full range of motion and no clicking or crepitus when the stifle is flexed and extended. No significant lameness is seen.

Grade 2 is frequent luxation, with self-realignment by the animal. Partial lameness on the affected limb is observed and range of motion is usually limited in the direction of bending. Pain and crepitus are seen in this grade category.

Grade 3 is frequent luxation that stays out of place and the animal cannot self-realign it. It can only be reduced manually by the therapist or veterinarian. The animal usually shows severe lameness with more weight shifted onto the front limbs during gait.

Grade 4 luxation exists when the patella is completely out of the groove and is not able to be realigned at all. Range of motion at the stifle joint is very limited and the animal typically walks in a crouched position with the limb partially bent.

The most common grades of patellar luxation that are seen in clinical practice are Grades 2 and 3. Grade 1 luxation does not require any treatment, just monitoring and veterinary examination during your annual visit. Grade 2 can greatly benefit from physical therapy treatment intervention. Grades 3 and 4 require surgery for correction and post-operative physical therapy. If these conditions are allowed to go untreated, irritation and chronic inflammation in the form of chondromalacia can develop over time.

The diagnosis is made by feeling or palpating the patella during physical examination, along with flexing and extending the stifle joint, and can be seen on radiograph (X-ray). It is not always necessary to have radiographs taken, unless the condition is severe and surgery is considered.

In terms of surgery, there are several methods to correct patellar luxation. A brief description of the four major types follows:

> Parapatellar release arthrotomy is a two-part procedure in which the soft tissues on the inner medial side of the stifle are cut, to release tautness, followed by a corresponding tightening on the outer lateral side. The medial structures that are released are the innermost band of the hamstrings (biceps femoris) and two front of the thigh muscles, which insert near the patella (sartorius and vastus medialis). A strip of the joint capsule on the outer lateral side of the stifle is loosened, overlapped, and sutured back down to tighten the opposite side. This is essentially a balancing procedure performed on the soft tissues.

> Wedge or block recession trochleoplasty is a surgical deepening of the groove that the patellar sits in. Special reaming devices are used to drill and reshape this canal, which is formed between the two bony knobs (trochlear condyles) found at the end of the femur.

> Transposition of the tibial tuberosity is another form of surgical procedure. The tuberosity of the tibia leg bone is a bump on which the thigh muscle is attached. This is

the quadriceps muscle that passes under and around the patella. With this technique, the tuberosity is removed and, carrying the muscle attachment and patella with it, is shifted slightly over toward the outer lateral side, then reattached. It is a relocation surgery, which provides a good angle in which the patella can stay in place when the quadriceps muscle contracts. Many times the surgeon will do this procedure along with the groove deepening trochleoplasty procedure above.

Corrective femur osteotomy is done on the thigh bone (femur) as opposed to the tibia in the leg. A wedge of femur bone is cut and removed on the side opposite to which the patella luxates. If the pet suffers from medial luxation, then the bone wedge will be taken off the lateral side. This wedge removal allows the surgeon to realign the angle of the long femur bone, so that the quadriceps muscle can pull the patellar in a better direction when it contracts.

After surgery, a padded bandage will be in place for a few days and the veterinarian will give you specific instructions regarding activity restriction. Physical therapy is likely to begin about two weeks post-op. The therapist will likely utilize cold packs and functional electrical stimulation to reduce swelling and begin to train the quadriceps muscle to work in a slightly altered direction, to help control the patella. Range of motion to bend and straighten the stifle will be applied carefully. Massage and gentle manual mobilization of the patella will be carefully performed to glide and stretch the tissues. Stretching the inner thigh muscles, hamstrings, and Achilles tendon will be included in treatment. The quadriceps muscle, however, should not be stretched at this time as it closely surrounds the patella and requires a period of healing after the surgery. Do not be afraid to ask the therapist to avoid stretching the quadriceps muscle during the initial weeks of recovery.

Strengthening will begin about three weeks after surgery using resistive bands tied around the rear limbs while the pet walks, along with other exercises such as sit to stand and walking through a tunnel. Walking in shallow water may also be beneficial. A Physio-Roll ball is often used by placing the front limbs over the ball with the animal bearing weight on the rear limbs, which are planted on the floor. The ball can gently be rolled back and forth to help the animal learn to shift its body weight back onto the rear limbs. The ball can also be repositioned to roll it from side to side, encouraging weight distribution onto the operated side. Leash walks can be started soon after surgery, for short distances such as three to five minutes. The distance and speed will be steadily increased over four to six weeks, and the therapist will include some turns, circle patterns, and side or backward stepping. You should not allow the pet to use steps or staircases during the first month after surgery.

If the pet has only a Grade 1 or 2 patellar luxation, thus not requiring any surgical intervention, it would be wise to ask the veterinarian to recommend physical therapy to help reduce the chances of the condition progressing. A typical session will involve laser to reduce inflammation, manual realignment of the patella, soft tissue stretching of structures on the tight side of the stifle, and strengthening of muscles and tendons on the loose side. This results in a rebalancing so that the patella is not pulled or allowed to drift off course within the trochlear groove. Some of these techniques are tricky and involve skill and experience to move the limb in three simultaneous dimensions, and fall into the "don't try this at home" category. Rest assured, however, that when properly and effectively performed, these techniques do not require multiple weeks of visits to the therapist. After a few sessions of realignment, you can be taught how to do some simpler, one-dimension stretching on a daily basis that will be very effective in maintaining stability of the patella.

Other problems that can occur with the patella are fractures and tendon ruptures. Patella fractures are uncommon and usually caused by direct trauma. The patellar tendon, which attaches the front thigh or quadriceps muscle to the tibia, can also rupture, causing the patella to ride upward. This situation requires surgery using tension wires to correct the positioning and fracture. Limited physical therapy may be helpful after several weeks of immobilization and rest, to help your pet regain range of motion of the stifle. Absolutely no quadriceps muscle stretching should be done at this time. In cases of fracture where the patella shattered and cannot be fixated, it is removed. This is called a patellectomy and is usually a last resort as it alters the normal walking mechanism.

Hock Injuries

Injuries to the animal hock or ankle are somewhat less common than with the hip and stifle joints, but they do occur and respond well to physical therapy. In dogs there are two likely scenarios that affect the hock: dropped hocks from weakness or tearing of the Achilles tendon, and slipped hocks from ligament instability.

Dropped hocks describe the abnormal position of the heels touching the ground in animals. As you already know from the basic anatomy section in Chapter 2, quadruped animals walk on their feet and digits, with the heels raised. When the hocks drop down, it is usually from either a birth defect or a torn or overstretched Achilles tendon. Achilles tendon tears are commonly seen in sporting dogs that race, hunt, and sled. The dogs will also have difficulty bearing weight on the affected limb. Surgery is often needed to repair the tendon along with bracing to support and stabilize the hock post-operation. Physical therapy typically begins four weeks after surgery with laser, ultrasound, massage, and range of motion. Depending on the surgeon's protocol, weight bearing, strengthening, and stretching will start at a later date as damage may occur if instituted too soon. Underwater treadmill walking is desirable as it provides a safe medium in which to begin gradually applying pressure to the repaired tendon. The use of balls and Physio-Rolls is helpful in placing the dog over to rock back and forth and start gently springing off the foot, thereby strengthening the calf muscles to elevate the hock. The final stages of therapy will focus on advanced strengthening with the use of rocker boards, walking up inclines and hind limb dancing forward and backward.

Slipped hocks display the opposite position of the dropped hock. Slipped hocks are hyperextended, with the heel elevated higher than normal and the foot pointing downward, similar to a ballerina's. You may even see the hock move forward in a rolling over unstable manner. This requires a veterinary consultation with possible surgery or hock splints, wraps, etc. After stability is gained, physical therapy is helpful in strengthening the shin or cranial tibia muscles.

Other hock conditions include sprains to the joint from trauma, falls, and jumps. I have treated many domestic cats with this injury and they respond rapidly to physical therapy. Common treatment sessions consist of laser, massage, range of motion, and regaining strength with climbing and bouncing on soft surfaces such as balance bubbles and Physio-Rolls. I have also provided treatment to birds having hock sprains, including a rooster named Galileo. Poor Galileo was hit by a car and survived. However, he had a bad bruise to his right leg and hock, and was unable to stand on it. Thus, he could stand only on one leg for brief periods, unable to walk or hop. His lovely owner refused to put him down and consulted a local animal sanctuary that referred her to a traveling veterinarian specializing in exotics, and then to me. He was an amazing patient, sweet and tolerant of my tucking his wings in and gently turning him on his side for laser, massage, and wrapping the joint for stabilization. Galileo eventually regained partial use of the leg and was able to stand and hop short distances. (See Note 12.)

Rotator Cuff

The rotator cuff in animals is somewhat different from that of humans, but both are designed to provide stability to the shoulder joint. Injury to the animal rotator cuff resulting in tears and instability is discussed later in Chapter 9, in the sports section. Here, we will look at another type of rotator cuff condition that involves one muscle in particular, the infraspinatus, and results in tightness and contracture. The cause is unknown but often seen in hunting injuries, or due to abnormal tension or forceful stress placed on the shoulder. I had an interesting example of this last summer when a new client contacted me about her geriatric Miniature Schnauzer, Louise, who had gone in for a dental procedure and came home with clean teeth but with a front leg that was hanging out! Trips back to the veterinarian and neurologist ruled out a stroke, but failed to determine a diagnosis. When the client sent me pictures of Louise by phone, it looked fairly obvious that the infraspinatus muscle was in a state of contracture. I need to clarify here, again, that we therapists do not formally diagnose patients, but can provide input based on our experience with conditions we commonly see in our practice. After a few quick communications, Louise started physical therapy for treatment of the contracture, thought to have possibly arisen from positioning and limb restraint during surgery. Another clarification: this is theory only and not any fault of the surgeon, as unexpected things can occur even when normal procedures are followed. We'll get back to Louise shortly.

The infraspinatus muscle, normally functioning as a lateral rotator (turning the shoulder outward), becomes hard and in a shortened state of contracture due to injury. The animal will hold the forelimb in an awkward position, with the elbow tucked in at its side while the forearm and paw are flipped outward while walking. In sitting or standing, the limb will be placed further away from the body than normal, with a visible indent on the shoulder blade. In many cases, the best treatment is a surgical release of the tight tendon bands and clearing of fibrotic scar tissue, followed by physical therapy. In other cases where surgery might be contraindicated for other medical reasons, or unaffordable, physical therapy is the only option. Laser or ultrasound, followed by deep friction massage and myofascial release technique is needed to break down fibrosis and scar tissue. Heat might also be used to increase blood flow to the area to provide muscle relaxation. Electrical stimulation in the form of NMES or FES can help provide a stimulus to artificially fatigue the muscle into a state of relaxation. All of this prepares the therapist to gently elongate the infraspinatus muscle and stretch it, gradually increasing range of motion. Further stretching can be achieved with a rocker board, placing the front paws on the board in symmetrical position and rocking the animal from side to side.

Now, back to Louise: having more surgery was not an option, so medication was prescribed for pain relief and muscle relaxation. Physical therapy was provided in the home with family members instructed in massage and stretching techniques to perform daily between therapy sessions. Louise gained sufficient pliability of the tendon with increased range of motion to be able to hold her limb closer to her side, not catching it in the doorway or tripping on the steps. This was further enhanced by the client building a ramp from the deck to the backyard. Best of all, she was now able to resume jumping up into grandma's lap for a good snuggle!

Elbow Fractures

Trauma is the usual culprit with fractures at or near the elbow in animals. Those occurring at the elbow are called "articular fractures" and are commonly at the end of the humerus bone. They occur less often at the radius and ulna. Elbow fractures need good repair and alignment, due to the critical weight-bearing function they provide for a quadruped animal. A veterinarian trained in orthopedic surgery will secure the alignment and congruity of the joint with the placement of screws and pins.

However, achieving post-fracture alignment is only part of the healing equation because without early physical therapy, decreased range of motion and bone or cartilage loss may occur. It is essential that your veterinarian show you how to start range of motion exercises at home or refer you to a qualified physical therapist to provide this service. Range of motion exercises must start within a few days to two weeks after the operation, depending on the surgeon's protocol, and continue daily for the first two to three weeks of rehabilitation. In particular, it is critical that elbow extension (straightening) be quickly regained. The use of cold packs, massage, medications, laser, and other interventions are included to improve motion and reduce pain and swelling. After the first three weeks of therapy, when adequate healing has been ascertained by the doctor, more intensive range of motion, stretching, and strengthening exercises can be initiated. The goal now is to rebuild atrophied musculature and progress to full weight bearing on the forelimb.

The second type of elbow fracture occurs a bit higher up from the actual joint, in the shaft of the humerus bone. Although most fractures that occur along the bone shaft are less complicated than those at the joint, this one is problematic because of the location of an important nerve that wraps around the humerus. It is called the radial nerve and is often compromised when a fracture occurs just above the elbow. The radial nerve controls the muscles that lift the front paw and straighten the elbow, so when there is radial nerve damage, your pet will begin to walk with a flipping action of the paw. No, they are not just being friendly and waving to you! They will be lame on one front limb, have difficulty bearing weight with the elbow unable to straighten fully, and the paw drooping as the leg is lifted. The initial physical therapy treatment for this is making a drop paw splint that can be worn during the day as the pet sits and walks, to hold it in place and prevent abrasion and further injury. The splint is usually worn for about six to eight weeks as the nerve heals. The therapist will remove the splint to examine the skin integrity, apply massage, and use NMES electrical stimulation to facilitate activation of the forearm muscles. When use of the splint can be discontinued, gait training with a leash and visual or touch commands can be started to help the pet regain control of the paw while walking.

Elbow Dysplasia

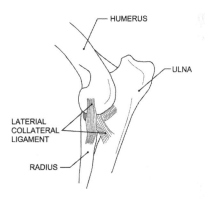

ELBOW

Figure 4

Do not confuse dysplasia of the elbow with that of the hip. It is entirely different. Hip dysplasia, as discussed earlier, is a type of laxity, but elbow dysplasia is a triad condition that develops into malformation and degeneration of this important weight-bearing joint. It is seen in large and giant breeds of dogs and appears to have genetic components in the way it manifests symptoms and signs. The three abnormalities of elbow dysplasia are:

1. FCP: Fragmented (medial) Coronoid Process. This condition has a genetic component and can become visible by radiograph in puppyhood. The medial coronoid process is located on the ulna, near the humerus, and along the inner side of the elbow. It is termed as "fragmented" due to the presence of spurs and bone degeneration.

2. OCD: Osteochondritis Dissecans. This condition affects the medial humeral condyle located at the inner side of the elbow, at the bottom of the humerus, where the bone forms rounded ends. The medical humeral condyle is located at the inner side of the elbow, at the bottom of the humerus, where the bone forms rounded ends. In this condition, the condyles become inflamed and have abnormal density of bone structure with degeneration.

3. UAP: Ununited Anconeal Process. The anconeal process, not present in humans, is a beak-like projection that is part of the ulna and located at the back or tip of the elbow. At birth, is has a normal crack or fissure that should close up around five months of age. Its purpose is to add stability for the animal's elbow as it is a weight-bearing joint. If it remains open after that, it generally stays that way and is called "ununited." If it is left untreated, the elbow does not match up correctly and swelling, pain, and bone erosion may take place, with eventual arthritis. UAP is seen more often in males than females. There is usually a gradual onset of lameness and limping and may not be noticed until later in life. (See Note 13.)

Most dogs diagnosed with elbow dysplasia have one of the above three conditions and rarely have all three. They generally have dysplasia in both elbows, but one is usually worse than the other. It is diagnosed by radiograph (X-ray) and clinical examination. Surgery is sometimes an option, performed with incisions along the back and outer border of the joint, to remove and excise bone spurs and abnormal growths. Arthroscopic surgery, done through a scope with tiny incisions, is the optimal choice as there are fewer traumas to the surrounding ligaments and joint capsule. Other treatment includes medications, supplements that support cartilage health, management of body weight, activity modification, and physical therapy. Typical physical therapy for elbow dysplasia consists of heat modalities, TENS for pain, laser, joint mobilization, range of motion exercises, controlled strengthening and low impact activity, swimming, underwater treadmill, and use of wraps and braces or other supports for the joint. Joint range of motion for elbow flexion and extension should be monitored and measured with a goniometer at regular intervals, to ensure that it is being maintained. Without good diagnosis and treatment planning, elbow dysplasia can lead to debilitating joint degeneration.

GREAT TO KNOW
"In 1990, OFA began its elbow dysplasia database. The number of OFA elbow valuations continues to increase significantly each year. This is a sign that there is growing awareness regarding elbow dysplasia and that breeders are seriously interested in reducing incidence of this disease."
Orthopedic Foundation for Animals (OFA)

Obviously, physical therapy cannot correct the underlying problems of elbow dysplasia, but can offer solutions to improve joint health and the animal's quality of life.

Carpus Hyperextension

If you've ever seen a dog, cat, or other small animal standing flat-pawed on its front limbs, you have witnessed carpus hyperextension. Quadrupeds, or animals that stand on four limbs, normally bear weight on the front digits and pads, with their carpus (wrist) joints raised up off the ground. When the supporting ligaments at the back of the carpus joints are torn, from a jumping or falling injury, there is disruption to these structures that normally provide lift. Occasionally, carpus hyperextension is seen in congenital defects of collagen, the protein substance that provides firmness to ligaments and other connective tissue. Surgical stabilization can be performed, but the majority of cases tend to be managed conservatively with physical therapy and splinting. I found success in the treatment of two canine carpus hyperextension cases: Natasha, a Husky mix, and Kermit, a Pit Bull-Hound mix, neither having surgery due to financial burden of their owners. Although some lifestyle changes were ultimately needed to manage the chronic instability, physical therapy provided partial correction of the condition. This was achieved through passive support of the joints via wraps and splints, and active control by strengthening the flexor tendons and muscles. FES electrical stimulation was done by placement of small electrodes on the under surface of the ante brachium (forearm), to contract the carpus flexor musculature for fifteen minutes. This was immediately followed by strengthening exercises using Thera Bands, playing with toys, tickling the flexor muscle bellies, bouncing on a Physio-Roll, and balancing on a rocker board. Outdoor walks in tall grass and sand provided a stimulus to high step and lift the carpus joints up. Treats were offered, being held overhead to encourage the dogs to rise upward on their toes. Pool swimming was used on the off therapy days to provide a fun, non-weight-bearing exercise alternative for joint protection and strength. Both patients were measured and fitted for custom carpus wraps of moderate fabric weight, to be worn during walks and active times of the day. They were removed for rest and fur/skin examined closely for any signs of wear or irritation. Eventually, the older of the two dogs had a molded splint fabricated by an occupational therapist, to replace the wrap in order to provide additional joint support. Both dogs needed close monitoring and long-term management of their weight, important to the front load-bearing carpus joints.

Fracture Luxation

Broken bones occurring along the middle of the shaft are relatively uncomplicated and usually do not require physical therapy. However, when bones break near their ends, a destruction to the joint, or luxation, occurs. These are also called "articular fractures," meaning that they occur where the bones meet and articulate at the joint. They can occur in dogs and other species of all ages, usually from some type of trauma, car accidents, jumping from heights, etc. I had one case involving a young Alaskan Huskie that jumped out of a second-story window, during one of our famous New Jersey nor-easters! These are common in the elbow, carpus, pelvis, and hips. Proper medical treatment and follow-up physical therapy is essential to prevent future development of bone spurs or fragments, bone loss, and arthritis. Surgery with internal fixation is often required, using wires, plates, and screws. Other times, external fixators are applied with careful management and cleaning of the pin sites to prevent infection. Physical therapy must be delayed typically for eight to twelve weeks to allow complete healing to occur. Electrical stimulation such as FES and NMES help with muscle building and strengthening, along with range of motion exercises and low impact activity such as swimming. When weight bearing can be resumed, leash walks must be short and progressed slowly, starting on softer surfaces such as grass initially.

A very unusual case involving a baby swan came my way last year. The little guy was found abandoned by his mother, likely after some sort of trauma, resulting in a broken heel and luxation/dislocation of the hock, near the junction of the web and digits. He was splinted and taped for a two-week period, during which time he received attentive care from zoo staff. Physical therapy began afterward using cold packs to the heel, laser, massage to the leg, and range of motion exercises for the hip, stifle, and hock. The greatest challenge was with the swan's webbed foot, which was weak and swollen. Initially the swan was unable to move the digits apart, spreading the web. Finally, the swelling subsided through rest, medication, and physical therapy modalities, resulting in partial recovery of strength and function. You can probably guess which method of strengthening exercise I chose for him: pool swimming, of course! Eventually he was able to walk, as swans do with their waddling, wheeling gait, with partial weight on the limb. Although I was happy for his recovery, I missed (and still miss) the precious way he wound his long neck around the back of mine as I held him against my chest and shoulder during treatment. He earned the name Snuggles because of that!

Brachial Plexus Injuries

The brachial plexus is a nerve center found near the animal's clavicle (or collarbone) at the pectoral region, which supplies innervation to the forelimb muscles. In animals, it can be injured by falls or incidents involving overstretch of the upper or front limb. An example is a cat jumping down from an elevated height and catching its paw on a shelf, or stretching up to investigate or swat an object and getting its paw stuck. Birds also are subject to brachial plexus injury if their neck is stretched or wing gets caught on a branch or wire. The result is a weak and flailing limb that drags while walking and collapses on attempts to bear weight, or the bird's inability to use its wing. In both cases, the poor animal is literally left hanging. Recovery varies depending on the degree of damage and species. Kittens with mild or partial brachial plexus injuries heal quickly and fully, whereas older cats recover at a slower rate. If the plexus is moderately damaged, recovery is very slow and with some residual weakness. Complete lesions of the plexus have a zero to minimal chance or recovery and amputation is often considered.

Here are two cases I had the opportunity to provide physical therapy for:

1. Nutella, a nine-week-old kitten: treatment consisted of laser therapy, range of motion, NMES electrical stimulation, weight bearing on an inflated balance bubble, and wheel-barrowing functional exercise. You might

be wisely noting that laser is not usually indicated for animals still growing, but in Nutella's case, it was her best option and would have been riskier to withhold it and delay proper healing. She recovered fully, in about six days!

2. Bobby, a Macaw parrot: he had severe wing damage with a humerus fracture and complete brachial plexus injury, resulting in amputation. Why did he need physical therapy? Bobby needed to regain balance and the ability to maneuver in his habitat effectively. He received massage, standing balance exercises, and adaptations to his living environment, including the addition of more tree branches with wide bridges between them to enable him to step safely and easily.

Bicep Tendonitis

You are likely to be familiar with the biceps or Popeye muscle in the human arm, also present in animals. The tendon of the biceps is a long, thick attachment that runs upward along the inner side of the humerus, at the front of the animal's shoulder. It becomes strained and inflamed because of hunting, agility, or racing activity, resulting in a condition of tendonitis. It can also be called "bicipital tenosynovitis." It is more common with middle-aged and medium to larger breeds of dogs such as Greyhounds, Dobermans, or Collies. It is difficult to diagnose with an X-ray and usually best determined by physical examination with two hallmark signs: tenderness to palpation of the tendon, in the inner or medial side of the upper humerus; and discomfort when the shoulder is flexed or stretched backward, with the animal's elbow straight. The animal will also limp, avoid stairs, walk slowly, and hold the affected forelimb in a flexed or protected position. Once diagnosed, bicep tendonitis is treated with activity restriction (jumping, running) for one to three months, injections, and physical therapy consisting of ice, ultrasound, laser, and transverse friction massage in a direction perpendicular to the tendon and muscle fibers, which would be across the arm, parallel to the floor. After the acute inflammatory phase, the therapist will begin stretching to the forelimb. If inflammation is severe and slow to resolve, a topical medication might be applied to the skin over the tendon, after shaving, prior to and during the application of ultrasound, called "phonophoresis." In the sub-acute phase of healing, strengthening begins using resisted Thera Bands, hurdle stepping, and controlled downward walking on ramps or inclined surfaces. If bicep tendonitis is not treated promptly or activity restriction isn't enforced, chronic inflammation with painful spurs or osteophytes can develop. The origin of bicep tendonitis is typically from overuse and repetitive movement, so cross-training with swimming or water walking is an excellent way to keep your pet conditioned without risk of tendon re-injury. It is also vitally important to listen to your veterinarian and physical therapist regarding their crucial advice on activity restriction and use of on leash only, controlled walking.

Congenital Anomalies

Unusual defects, present at birth, are seen in organ, skin, and musculoskeletal systems. Some resolve as the animal grows, but many result in permanent structural changes that the animals must live with and adapt to. This section will address those anomalies that affect bones and joints of individual animals and that are not considered to occur from genetic diseases. They are generally termed "somatic mutations," or those that do not involve the reproductive germ cells, and therefore not passed on to the next generation. The factors that might cause such defects in single patients are: environment, trauma, infection, diet and nutrition, toxins and chemicals, birth injuries, and chromosome aberrations.

Physical therapists working with animals are often called on to help those patients with congenital anomalies achieve symptom relief and maximum functioning.

Here are three examples of defects that benefit from physical therapy intervention:

1. Transitional vertebrae is an extra vertebrae that is poorly formed with an unusual shape, and typically found at the bottom of the spine, just below the last lumbar vertebra. Its presence causes irritation and compression of the tail section of the spinal cord and spinal nerves, and is called "Cauda Equina syndrome" (CES). One of the hallmark signs of this is a limp tail. Other signs include loss of control of the hind limbs with muscle wasting and bowel and/or bladder incontinence. This condition worsens as the animal ages. It is diagnosed with radiographs and neurological clinical examination. It is treated with medications, surgery (in some cases), and physical therapy for modalities to relieve discomfort and strengthening of the core and hind limb musculature. Assistance with adaptive equipment such as standing harnesses, slings, and wheeled walkers or carts can also be provided.

Pet owners should be instructed in range of motion exercises for the rear limbs and massage to the lower spine to perform at home several times per week.

2. Atlanto-Axial (AA) luxation is another type of spine anomaly, but it occurs higher, in the neck region. The top two neck vertebrae—atlas (first cervical) and axis (second cervical)—are formed distinctly different from the rest of the spinal column. Their pairing results in the side-to-side rotation of the upper neck, similar to the movement of a person shaking his or her head "no." This head-turning movement relies on good stability normally provided by a finger-like bony projection on the axis, called "dens," and surrounding ligaments. When a birth defect of the dens exists, such as a fractured or missing dens, the result is instability or luxation. Clinical signs of this usually present themselves within the first weeks of life and can result in spinal cord trauma affecting all four limbs and the trunk. I had a fascinating case involving Timmy, a tiny Dachshund-Chihuahua mix, who was found in the presence of a kind, homeless man in Miami, Florida. Timmy, adorable but unable to walk, caught the eye of an avid runner jogging along the street who adopted him and provided for his every need. Blood work, radiographs, myelogram, and spinal tap confirmed the suspected AA luxation. Timmy received medication for inflammation, gastrointestinal protection, and pain, followed by surgery a few days later to place screws and pins with bone cement to reduce and stabilize the joint. Physical therapy began twelve weeks after surgery with FES electrical stimulation, massage, and extensive

strengthening to the spinal and limb musculature using Thera Bands, manual resistance, Physio-Rolls, donut bubble, rocker board, plus functional exercises and controlled leash walking. Because Timmy was still very much a puppy, leash walks were vital to slow his pace and force him to use the limb musculature correctly. Without this, Timmy would have simply bunny hopped and placed most weight distribution onto the front limbs, with his spine curved up in a roached posture. Timmy did beautifully with this therapy and loving care from his adoptive parents, regaining significant strength and the ability to walk and run.

3. Angular limb deformity occurs mainly in the forelimbs from abnormalities of the growth plates in the distal parts of the radius and ulna. This produces a twisting and bowed appearance of the carpus (wrist) joints, called "varus." It can also produce the opposite, or a knocked knee luxation of the carpus called "valgus." Either direction is abnormal and if untreated, can result in future arthritis for an animal. Surgery is available consisting of corrective cutting and resetting of the bones with internal plates or external fixation devices. Other dogs do not have this surgery for a variety of reasons, including Samsonite, an eight-year-old brindled Cane Corso Italian Mastiff I encountered at an animal shelter. He had been living with this deformity all of his life and limped during walking, with only partial weight on the carpus. He received physical therapy with ultrasound, massage, and gentle range of motion of the carpus joints with manual elongation technique toward the normal

neutral direction that would have been available if the anomaly had not occurred. In other words, I could not correct the angle, but I could allow a temporary respite for the joint through applying these distraction stretch techniques. Samsonite was eventually able to walk comfortably with nearly full weight on the carpus joints. He was a lovely affectionate boy who found a permanent home with a young couple in Rhode Island.

Wounds

Many of the modalities used in physical therapy are helpful in wound healing. Lasers, electrical stimulation, and massage increase blood flow to the wound and enhance cell metabolism to facilitate recovery. Physical therapists receive training in the care of wounds and burns as part of their professional education. Animals receive wounds from bites, trauma, surgery, abrasion injury, lacerations, punctures, burns, as well as skin ulcerations and lick granulomas. Some of these can prove difficult to heal, require lengthy treatments, and be at risk for infection. The veterinarian, while providing the overall medical management, may seek additional assistance from a physical therapist to help speed up the healing process. The initial acute stage of wound care includes medications for pain, inflammation, and infection, prescribed by the veterinarian, plus cleaning, bandaging, confinement, and activity restriction. This stage usually lasts two to three days. As the wound starts the next stage of repair, debridement is performed by the doctor or therapist, using scalpel, scissors and forceps, gauze, or chemicals to carefully and gently remove dead or damaged tissue, to promote healing and growth of healthy tissue. This stage usually begins on the third to fifth day, and lasts until two to four weeks after surgery or injury. If the wound or burn is deep, also called "full thickness," a red lumpy granulation tissue starts to grow as the healing begins. If the wound is not as deep, called "partial thickness," a pink epithelial tissue will be seen. The final stage is maturation, which starts after fourteen to twenty days and lasts varying amounts of time, depending on the medical condition and type of care rendered. During this stage, scar tissue develops and final closure occurs.

At this point, physical therapy will consist of scar mobilization and massage, likely cross friction methods, range of motion, and stretching exercises. Various wound ointments or salves might be used such as antibiotic creams, silver sulfadiazine (Silvadene), aloe vera, and vitamin E gel that your therapist can help you administer. (See Note 14.)

Sprains and Strains

They sound similar, but are distinctly different! A sprain refers to a ligament that has been overstretched and injured. Ligaments are the strong, thick fibrous bands that connect bone to bone, holding joints together. An example of this is the cranial cruciate ligament (CCL) that is injured, but not torn. It might be overstretched and inflamed, but if not actually torn, it would be considered a sprain.

Strains refer to injuries affecting muscles and tendons. Tendons are the tough bands that connect muscle to bone. An example of this is the biceps tendon in the shoulder. It can be pulled and twisted, resulting in pain and inflammation, resulting in a strain.

Both sprains and strains occur from slips, falls, jumps, twists and turns, running, etc. The animal will usually show symptoms of yelping or crying, tenderness, warmth, and lameness. The veterinarian will diagnose sprains and strains mainly by physical examination, including feeling or palpating the injury site, moving the joints and limbs, and taking radiographs to rule out fractures or other injuries. Sprains and strains are not visible on radiograph (X-ray).

The key to healing sprains and strains is early diagnosis and treatment. Although this might sound obvious, some pet owners avoid a trip to the doctor right after the injury occurs, adopting a wait-and-see approach. This is tempting, as sprains and strains do not present as dramatically as a bone fracture or wound might. The best advice is to get an injury checked out early, even if it doesn't seem severe, as soft tissues can be slow to heal if not treated promptly. You know the saying "it's better to break a bone"…!

Treatment includes rest, medication, wraps, or other types of support or immobilization, use of laser, cold packs, ultrasound, etc. After the acute phase, massage, range of motion, stretching, and gradual return to activity are implemented, on the advice of your doctor or therapist.

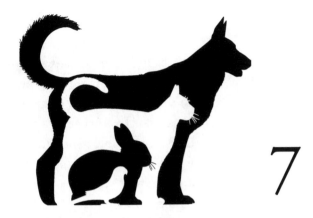

7

Rehabilitation of Neurological Conditions

Degenerative Myelopathy

When faced with a particularly difficult challenge in life, I have always felt the best weapon of combat is knowledge. Along with that is keeping a positive attitude. As a physical therapist, dealing with canine patients diagnosed with degenerative myelopathy is both rewarding and heart wrenching. Keeping dog parents informed and equipped with management tools is essential to optimization of the condition.

Degenerative myelopathy (DM) is a painless, chronic, slowly progressive weakening starting in the hind limbs and lumbar region. There is diffuse muscle atrophy (wasting), the paws begin to knuckle under, the legs drag with a loss of coordination, and walking becomes very difficult. It tends to progress over five to six months. It is most common in certain breeds of dogs such a German Shepherds, Welsh Corgis, Chesapeake Bay Retrievers, Boxers, Collies, and Rhodesian Ridgebacks. It typically appears between seven and fourteen years of age. The diagnosis is by exclusion in ruling out other causes. Radiographs (X-rays) will be negative for dysplasia, IVDD, arthritis, or tumors. In the near future, the diagnosis may be more definitive through the emergence of a blood test that detects genetic markers for the condition. OFA may be able to provide some DNA testing information for you, your breeder, and veterinarian.

DM is quite similar to multiple sclerosis in human beings. Some dogs experience a form of it similar to ALS (Lou Gehrig's disease), which includes loss of function of the cranial nerves that control swallowing, facial movements, etc. The cause is unknown, although recent research has found a possible genetic link through a mutated gene. The mechanism is non-inflammatory and demyelinating (stripping) of the nerves in the spinal cord. DM is thought to be autoimmune in origin whereby the immune system attacks the myelin sheath. This is the outer covering of nerves, like insulation over electrical wires, so when it is stripped or covered in plaques, the nerve communication is decreased (similar to when your computer slows down because of noise on your cable).

The bad news is that at the present time there is no cure for DM. The good news is that the disease is not painful for the dog and is generally harder on the dog parents than the dog. There are many decisions that have to be made at various stages of the disease regarding the dog's and the family's maximum quality of life. If the family stays involved in the decision process, and can provide the best possible canine care, the dog will generally stay content and happy. I can't stress enough the importance of a commitment from the family. Because DM is a difficult condition to manage, it is best shared by various family members who form a care-giving team. For older members, it can provide a routine and fulfillment. For younger family members and kids, it can build responsibility. If everyone pitches in, the workload will be less and the dog will feel like a superstar. The family will also need a reality check as to goals, and be prepared to face regression.

There is help for these dogs and their families. The following is a list of my top ten suggestions for management of DM:

1. Specialty regional veterinary hospitals can be considered to provide inpatient care, diagnostic tests, and rehabilitation services to initially maximize the dog's condition and formulate a home treatment plan, order equipment, etc.

2. If inpatient care is too expensive or not available, many veterinary facilities now offer rehabilitation services as an outpatient. There are also independent canine rehab practitioners/physical therapists who offer care in their offices or in your home. Rehab should include an evaluation, intervention using range of motion, stretching, massage, gentle strengthening using resisted bands, Physio-Rolls, rocker boards, sensory input techniques, sling-assisted walking, etc. Some physical modalities such as electrical stimulation may be used. Aquatic therapy is also very helpful and important in maintaining mobility via canine swimming pool programs or underwater treadmills. Water buoyancy can benefit walking; standing and swimming should be done in short bouts.

3. Your vet can help you learn about bowel and bladder management, manual bladder expression, keeping a schedule, cleaning your dog, checking for soiling or urine scalding. Sometimes shaving the region is used to prevent infections.

4. Consider using a padded and possibly elevated dog bed for comfort and ease of on/off. Help your dog with frequent turning to avoid pressure sores.

5. Bring the dog outdoors and keep it moving, but avoid over exertion, heat, and limit its exposure to sun.

6. Slings and harnesses assist the dog transferring from lying to sitting, to standing, during walking, and while turning.

7. Identify and avoid barriers in the home such as stairs or uneven floors and reduce slippery surfaces by adding carpet runners or non-skid mats.

8. Routinely check the dog's skin for scrapes or sores, infections, abnormal wear of nails, and pads. Booties are available for foot protection when the hind limbs drag and also offer anti-slip control. Consult your vet, PT, and groomer for suggestions.

9. Ask the vet or other pet expert about proper nutrition, protein consumption, hydration, and weight management. Help with the dog's ability to use food and water bowls by positioning them close, on a non-skid pad, and at proper height.

10. Wheeled carts can be helpful for your dog's mobility. Standard rear-wheeled carts are fine if the forelimbs are strong. If the rear legs show knuckling, the feet and hocks need to be supported by a sling or stirrup in the back of the cart. In many other cases, especially where the trunk and forelimbs become weakened, a counterbalanced cart is more effective, starting with neutral and progressing to full counterbalancing (this refers to a forward shift in the axle position). Some companies offer a variable axle, which can be adjusted by the dog

owner. Engineering, quality, and workmanship are so important when choosing a company to make the cart. I highly recommend Eddie's Wheels in Massachusetts.

Intervertebral Disc Disease of the Spine

Injuries and diseases that affect the discs of the spine (IVDD) are quite dramatic and disabling. This supportive column of bone, which encases the nerve centers of communication to and from the brain, provides a vital role in daily function for all animals. Canines can be affected by spinal conditions from the neck to the middle and lower sections of the spine. The dog breeds that are most prone to mid- and lower-spine problems are the dwarf, or "chondrodystrophic "body types, having short, bowed limbs. Examples are the Dachshund, Pekingese, Lhasa Apso, Corgi, and Basset Hound. Their spinal columns are proportionally longer in length, due to the disparate limb size, causing stress and strain.

Discs are spacers and shock absorbers, placed between each of the bony vertebrae. They are round structures with outer walls that consist of cartilage rings, similar to those of a tree trunk, with a soft jelly-like interior. The outer wall is called the "annulus fibrosis" and the inner substance is the "nucleus pulposus." The spinal column needs the discs as spacers to provide room for the nerves that branch off the spinal cord to exit. It also needs the discs as shock absorbers to protect and shield these nerves from jolts and stress.

Discs become injured when they are weakened and result in a bulge or rupture, causing irritation to the nerve. The weakening is caused by external pressures from tumors, poor posture, weight gain, loss of muscle tone and support, bone spurs, etc.

It can also occur from trauma or twisting/turning injuries, which crack the outer walls of the disc and cause the inner pulp to break through to the outside. If the damage is minor, the discs will simply bulge, but not break open. If this is treated promptly, the bulge usually resolves and the disc returns to its normal shape. When the damage is more significant, the disc will rupture and cause significant pain and irritation to the spinal nerves.

The canine spine, like the human, consists of three sections: cervical (neck), thoracic (ribs and middle section), and lumber (lower back). Both dogs and humans have seven cervical verte-brae, but the dog has one more thoracic and two more lumbar vertebrae. Thus, a dog has seven cervical, thirteen thoracic, and seven lumber vertebrae. Eighty percent of intervertebral disc injuries occur between the first thoracic and the third lumbar vertebrae.

Here is how most veterinarians classify disc disease:

Type 1: a total rupture of the outer wall, or annulus fibrosis, with massive break-through herniation of the inner nucleus pulposus. There is a sudden, acute onset of pain with neu-rological signs. Bowel and bladder functioning may be impaired. Neurological signs are moderate weakness in the rear limb; loss of coordination; severe weakness or paralysis in the rear limb; diminished sensation of the ability to feel hot/cold, sharp/dull, or deep pressure stimulus; numbness or tingling; abnormal reflexes. The dog will move slowly, drag one or both rear limbs, be reluctant or unable to jump, have a hunched or roached topline posture, and the tail may be limp. The dog may be unable to stand or be very unsteady on the rear legs.

Type 2: a partial rupture, with gradual onset of symptoms. There is pain but no, or very minor, neurological symptoms. Disc bulges also fall into this category. Disc bulges can present with a sudden onset of pain but only for a short period of a few hours to one day.

Mild cases of intervertebral disc disease such as Type 2 can be successfully treated conservatively with rest and medications (typically corticosteroids). This can include actual cage rest or reduced activity. Physical therapy can begin after the acute phase is over, in about five days.

More serious cases such as Type 1 may need surgery, such as hemilaminectomy (thoracic-lumbar region) or dorsal decompression laminectomy (lumbar and sacral region). Expect further testing such as an MRI or myelogram before surgery is recommended so that the extent and level of disc injury can be determined. Hemilaminectomy is a surgical technique approached from the side of the vertebrae and uses drilling with a burr apparatus to remove a portion of bone called the laminae. This provides more opening for the nerve and decompresses it. The surgeon also removes any extruded disc material that is pressing on the nerve. The dorsal decompression technique is similar but approached from the top or backside of the vertebrae. These surgeries are usually performed by veterinary specialists such as neurologists or orthopedists.

Many pet owners are reluctant to proceed with surgery and may seek alternative treatments. This is a highly personal decision and should be made after obtaining information, possible risks, and benefits along with a prediction of prognosis. One of the most important indicators of prognosis is the presence or absence of deep pain sensation in the rear limb and whether bowel and bladder functioning is present. If deep pain sensation is absent and there is no control of bowel or bladder for more than a few days, the chances of good functional recovery may be limited. Your surgeon can provide more information to assist your decision. You will also want to take into consideration the dog's lifestyle and how they might cope with a change toward more sedentary, house pet living if the results of disc disease are irreversible.

Cervical disc disease, occurring in the dog's neck, is the second most common form of intervertebral disc problems. It can be caused by trauma, rough neck movements from hard play or sports activity, or from degenerative conditions. The chondrodystrophic breeds mentioned above are affected by cervical disc problems, but in addition, larger breeds such as Great Danes, Dobermans, Mastiffs, etc., are affected as well. Larger breeds, especially those at middle to senior ages, can develop degenerative discs that settle, like an old house into the ground, which causes vertical pressure on the disc and irritation to the nerves called "radiculitis." Other degenerative spinal conditions include spondylosis, which is a narrowing condition with spurs and osteophytes that cause nerve pressure and radiating pain with weakness, called "radiculopathy." The most common signs are muscle atrophy, lameness on one or both of the front limbs, neck pain and stiffness, rigid and stiff muscles in the neck area, described as spasm. The dog may hold the front limbs very straight and wide apart in stance. The dog can also circle in pain, pant, have difficulty lying or sitting down, and hold its head in a down-facing position. These cases are usually treated conservatively at first, with corticosteroids, muscle relaxers, and pain and anti-inflammatory medications. If surgery is needed, the method used is a ventral slot technique and is approached from the front or underside of the vertebrae to remove bone and disc material for decompression of the nerve root.

Physical therapy treatment begins after a prescribed period of post-operative healing, based on the veterinary surgeon's instruction, which is usually at least two weeks. Some dogs stay in the veterinary hospital one to two days before returning home. Good care is needed in the early days following surgery for bowel and bladder management, and positioning and turning to prevent ulcers of the skin or urine scalds. You will receive detailed instructions from the surgeon that must be followed exactly. When the dog returns for suture removal, the surgeon will determine when physical therapy is safe to begin. Rehabilitation typically begins with laser to fully seal the incision and reduce unneeded scar tissue, electrical stimulation for pain relief or to facilitate muscle strengthening, massage, range of motion of the limbs, and home exercise instructions for you and the family to follow, between sessions. As soon as possible, the dog can begin standing and balance with weight-shifting exercises, functional activities such as sit to stand, and slow walking with harness and leash. Limb and core body strengthening exercises are an essential part of therapy, using propping cushions, limb weight bearing over a bolster, Physio-Rolls or balls, foam rolls, underwater treadmills, pool swimming, etc.

If there is significant weakness and debilitation, a sling around the belly can be used for support and assistance with standing and walking. In cases where the sensation is impaired, the dog may not feel if it is dragging its legs, and scrapes or abrasions along the top portion of the paw can occur. The therapist should caution you about this and recommend assistive devices to avoid abrasions that can potentially become infected.

Devices can range from rubber toe grippers to traction booties, supportive wraps or splints, or pull-up stockings, depending on the level of weakness or paralysis. When the dog has paralysis or diffuse weakness and is unable to walk, a wheeled cart should be considered. The therapist can guide you in researching the products and taking accurate measurements.

For the milder cases that do not require surgery, physical therapy can begin right away and include more aggressive methods and techniques such as spinal joint mobilization and manipulation, manual traction to the neck or lumbar regions, muscle stretching, active neck extension exercises encouraging the dog to look up, rolling activities, core stabilization, and tail pull releases, all performed by a trained therapist.

Here are two cases I had the pleasure of handling, one that needed surgery and one that did not.

First is Zoey, an eight-year-old female Pekingese, who underwent a lumbar hemilaminectomy for a herniated disc at the L3 (lumbar third vertebrae) in late March 2010. After a healing period of five weeks, physical therapy began in May, as advised by the neuro veterinary surgeon. Zoey's incision was healing well, her appetite and bowel/bladder function returned to normal. She was unable to sit up or stand on her own volition and required maximal assistance to be placed in these positions. Her left hind limb was weak and the right fully paralyzed. She was unable to walk and scooted herself throughout the house on her rump using the front legs, with the rear limbs dragging underneath. Deep reflexes were present but decreased, and sensation only partially present. In speaking to the family, I learned that Zoey was a very active dog that loved car rides and outings to the boardwalk at the Jersey Shore as well as taking long walks on paved trails. It was pretty obvious that this was not a dog that would be satisfied with house- and yard-confined sling walking. Because she loved being out in the community, we quickly determined that a wheeled cart would be the best option for these outings. We measured Zoey for a cart, sent in the form, and got to work with her therapy program. I used functional electrical stimulation with electrodes placed over the spinal musculature on each side of the surgical incision, as well as over weakened muscles of the left hind leg. I wanted to focus initially on the areas of greatest potential, to give her the ability to stand and sit independently, before addressing the paralyzed right hind leg. Massage and laser were applied to the surgical area, range of motion given to the rear limbs, stretching for tightness of the Achilles tendons, and placement of Zoey over a small Physio-Roll to elongate her spine and allow her limbs to bear weight while being supported. Muscle tone began to improve and Zoey was able to pull herself up to a sitting position within two weeks. By four weeks, Zoey could stand in one place, after being assisted into position, and maintain her balance for ten seconds. I began to shift the electrode placement to the paralyzed right hind limb, while advancing treatment to the left with resisted Thera Bands. By this time, Zoey could easily stand independently, but was still unable to walk. For in-house locomotion, she scooted on the floor with the front limbs and some pushing from the left hind limb. Due to the right limb dragging, we ordered a pull-on protective sock to prevent abrasion. A sling assist was used to help Zoey walk on three limbs outdoors in the yard to relieve her bowels and bladder. A rubber mat was placed under Zoey's food bowls to elevate them and help provide support while she stood.

Zoey's wheeled cart arrived, from Eddie's Wheels, amid much excitement from the family and a bit of anxiety from me (we therapists are always a bit nervous until we see that our careful measurements yield a good fit!). The cart was beautifully built and fit Zoey perfectly! Once applied, she needed only a few seconds of training before she learned to propel herself easily using the front limbs. Turns and corners needed a bit of practice but she soon mastered them and sped along, with her rear limbs safely protected from dragging and scrapes. Zoey was never able to walk on her own, but she loves her cart and rolls along the boardwalk every weekend, amid admiring glances and smiles from passers-by.

The next case is an adorable Dachshund-Chihuahua mix, named Cleopatra, age seven. Cleo had a lower lumbar partially herniated disc, as viewed by MRI. This was considered a Type 2 intervertebral disc disease, so surgical intervention was not considered. The dog's owners confided in me that they would not have been willing to try surgery anyway, based on their personal belief system of preferring holistic medicine. I explained that physical therapy was based on Western, traditional medicine but they were fully accepting of it as an alternative to surgery. A short course of oral prednisone was given, to provide rapid resolution of inflammation. Tramadol and Gabapentin were also prescribed by the veterinarian for pain relief. Cleo was a bit overweight and stood with a rounded topline, hind limbs tucked underneath so that she stood in a crouched position. Both hind limbs were weak, especially the left, but she had partial active control of each. She was able to stand but could not walk without the assistance of a sling. During walking, her right hind limb was full weight bearing, but the left was partial and lacked control at the distal end, where knuckling occurred. Deep tendon reflexes and balance were good. Cleo flinched when I attempted to palpate, or feel her spinal muscles in the lumbar region. She had full sensation to deep pain but her tail did not wag and was flaccid. I asked about the type of bed used for sleeping and was told that Cleo slept on the furniture, given freedom to jump on and off at will. My first order of business was to eliminate the jumping and use a crate while the parents were at work. When they were home, I asked them to block access to the furniture with boxes and pillows. Eventually a small ramp was built so Cleo could walk up to her favorite sofa. Laser and massage were used to relieve pain, muscle spasm, and tenderness along the lumbar spine. Joint mobilization of Grade 2 was applied with my hands along tight areas of the spine, along with elongation and stretching over a small Physio-Roll. Resisted exercises and gentle bouncing on an inflated bubble helped with strengthening the rear limbs. Core muscle strengthening was administered on a floor mat with Cleo on her back and side, along with light resisted rolling. As she gained strength and relaxation of muscle spasm, we began standing balance and weight-shifting exercises and gait training using the sling.

I advised Cleo's parents to discuss diet modification with their veterinarian for achieving some weight loss. Within three sessions, Cleo stopped knuckling on the left hind limb during her walks and we were able to wean use of the sling by the sixth visit. Cleo's walks were limited to non-slip surfaces such as carpet and grass. Once she stopped knuckling, we added the outdoor sidewalk. Cleo's posture became less guarded and her walking speed increased, along with distance. By this time, she had weaned off from the corticosteroids and used pain medication only intermittently. Cleo eventually was able to walk with a harness and leash in the neighborhood for seven to ten minutes twice per day. She could climb easily up and down two to three steps, but was carried up and down full staircases to prevent injury to her spine. Cleo was formally discharged from physical therapy after six weeks, but her mom calls me every few months for a few tune-up visits of spinal massage, joint mobilization, and manual spinal traction to keep pressure off the disc and help maintain Cleo's improvement.

Prevention of disc disease as well as recurrence is vitally important for your dog and the family. Here are my top ten tips for helping to avoid strain on spinal discs:

1. Avoid the use of traditional dog collars. Choose a supportive chest and thoracic harness for leash walking, hiking, and trotting.

2. Use a rolled towel or round pillow placed under the curve of your dog's neck when it is resting. It might not want to sleep with it but will tolerate it during naps and snuggle time with you and the family. Choose a size that matches the curve of the neck and is not oversized. If the dog has lumbar, or low back problems, place a folded-over towel or flat pillow under its belly when lying on the stomach, or placed between the thighs if side lying.

3. Maintain a reasonable, lean weight for your dog, as advised by the veterinarian.

4. Avoid dog doors that require your pet to push it open using its nose or head. Unless it is very easy to push, this activity can put pressure on the cervical discs.

5. Use ramps instead of steps for negotiating inclines. Avoid jumping on/off furniture by blocking the area or using a small ramp.

6. Consider using soft cervical collar supports intermittently if your dog has moderate arthritis and degenerative disc disease of the neck. These can be ordered from pet

brace companies and worn off and on throughout the day to reduce jarring and irritation to the disc and spinal joints. These are different from immobilization collars, which are used in cases of instability.

7. Keep food and water bowls elevated to a proper height to avoid excessive neck flexion, which places pressure on the cervical discs if the dishes are low on the floor. On the other hand, you want to avoid raising bowls too high, which might pinch a nerve if bone spurs or arthritis are present. There is also a risk of air-intake causing bloat from eating or drinking from bowls placed too high, especially in the deep-chested dogs such as Boxers. The best rule to follow in determining height elevation is when your dog is standing and eating or drinking, its head should be in a straight line from its withers, or dipped just slightly below. If you were to place a vertical ruler extending straight out from the withers, the top of your dog's head should be just under it, bent down no more than 25 degrees. Remember that the withers is the highest part of the dog's shoulders, at the base, or bottom of the neck. So, you might have to purchase several stands to find the optimal height and return the others. For large breeds the heights usually range from twelve to sixteen inches from the floor, medium sizes six to ten inches, and small or toy breeds three to six inches.

8. Place a non-skid cushioned thin mat for your dog to stand on while eating and drinking. This provides limb control and takes the strain off the discs, generated by standing in one place on a hard floor.

9. Avoid heavy twisting, head shaking, or tugging movements during play. Some folks feel that tug of war is

never a good mode of play for medical and behavioral reasons. I don't necessarily agree with that but if your dog has a known spinal issue, I would avoid these types of play activities or keep their duration short and seldom!

10. If your budget can afford, it may be wise to see a chiropractor or physical therapist, animal-trained of course, for some preventative joint manipulations, mobilizations, traction, and core strengthening exercises, on a monthly basis. (See Note 15.)

Instability/Wobbler Syndrome

Aptly named for its characteristic wobbly, uncoordinated gait, Wobbler syndrome is a condition that affects large breed animals. Its formal medical name is caudal cervical spondylopathy, affecting the lower neck vertebrae: C5, C6, and C7. It is caused by abnormal anatomical formations in the cervical spine, which cause the neck to be unstable, with pressure and compression upon the spinal cord. The result is pain and neurological problems: floating, high-step pattern of walking at the front limbs, clumsiness in the hind legs, awkward low carriage of the head, poor balance, loss of muscle tone, weakness. Wobbler syndrome has a hereditary component and progressively worsens over time. In dogs, it is usually seen in Great Danes and Doberman Pinschers. Some veterinarians advocate spinal surgery to stabilize the cervical spine and others use a conservative approach without surgery. Either way, physical therapy can offer some comfort and support for animals afflicted with Wobbler syndrome.

Due to the unstable nature of Wobbler syndrome, I will start by stating what should NOT be done in physical therapy:

there should be no use of passive range of motion exercise, joint mobilization, joint manipulation, stretching involving movement of any kind at the neck or thoracic spine. There are some traction techniques that are helpful for dogs with Wobbler's, performed with the neck in slightly flexed, bent forward position, but only a therapist or veterinarian can determine which dogs are appropriate for it. Dog collars should be avoided and replaced by harnesses. A soft-molded neck brace or support is usually recommended for use during therapy, walks, and upright activity. A human whiplash-style collar brace can be used for some dogs. Electrical stimulation in the form of TENS for pain control and/or FES for increase of muscle tone may be applied as well as laser, soothing massage techniques, and applying heat or cold packs. Exercises to strengthen the spine and limb muscles are important but must be done in a very specific way by the therapist: initially the flexor muscles that bend the neck forward will be given focus. The opposite muscle group, extensors that tilt the head back, will be gradually added into the exercise program, but only within a safe range of motion, as determined by the therapist. If the head and neck are allowed to bend too far backward, it may result in pain and spinal cord damage. Exercises to strengthen the limb muscles will also be performed, with the animal in a "stable," supported position over a bolster or Physio-Roll. Swimming and aqua therapy is sometimes recommended for Wobbler's but I tend to refrain from using pools and suggest using an underwater treadmill instead. It can be difficult to provide stability of the cervical spine and overall control of the dog having Wobbler's in a large open pool. The contained, enclosed space of the underwater treadmill provides a more stable environment with the opportunity for walking with partial weight limb contact. On land, walking distance and length of time should be limited to reduce excess stress on the spine. Some veterinarians prescribe periods of crate rest during the day for this purpose. Wheeled carts can be considered for use in Wobbler's but they must be modified to reduce strain on the neck and front limbs. Instead of a typical two-wheeled cart, quad or four-wheeled carts are usually a better choice in weight distribution and de-loading of the front limbs. Once a dog is non-ambulatory, a wagon-style device provides an option for letting your pet enjoy an outing with the family.

Stroke and Seizures

Cerebral vascular accident (CVA) or stroke is a rare event in animals. It is an interruption of blood supply to the brain caused by blood clot, tumor, or hemorrhage. Medical conditions such as Cushing's, diabetes, kidney, and heart disease can also affect circulation and lead to stroke. Although rare, it is seen and treated by physical therapists after the medical event is stabilized. Symptoms of stroke include weakness of the limbs on one side of the body, loss of bowel and bladder control, loss of consciousness, and walking in circles in one particular direction. This one-sided weakness is called "hemiparesis" and when there is actual paralysis it is "hemiplegia." It should also be noted that when weakness is present on one side, the forelimb is typically worse than the hind limb. There may also be increased motor tone with tightness in the muscles and shaking or tremors. Physical therapy can be helpful in relaxing tone in the limbs, stretching tight or spastic muscles, and preserving range of motion. Therapeutic exercises to facilitate movement and gain strength by stroking and tapping the muscles can be helpful. Balance and weight-shifting exercises are used to improve walking. Splints or wraps can be recommended to help control and support the weakened limbs, especially if the paws are dragging. A cheerful approach and positive attitude by the treating therapist and family members is essential for the animal's recovery.

Prognosis after stroke is varied, but the earlier rehabilitation is started, the more likely an animal is to improve. Early interventions help to form new nerve pathways in the brain through neuroplasticity. The neuroplasticity theory is gaining prominence in the physical therapy and rehabilitation professions. Certain high-profile cases involving traumatic brain injury such as the Arizona shooting incident involving Congresswoman Gabrielle Giffords and her subsequent rehabilitation have brought widespread attention to this theory. It applies to animal rehabilitation methods as well. The idea is that the central nervous system has the ability to adapt its chemical organization and structure in response to variable internal and external stimuli. The nervous system encodes the experiences met during therapy and relearns new behaviors in response to rehabilitation. While the animal is learning new patterns of movement and gaining the ability to balance and take independent steps, the therapist and pet owner should monitor the animal for signs of stress such as vomiting, panting, drooling, or drowsiness, and adjust treatment accordingly.

Seizures, different from stroke, are abnormal bursts of electrical activity in the brain. Physical therapy is not used to treat seizures but I have chosen to mention it in this book as it is highly important for the therapist to be aware if your pet has a seizure disorder. If an animal that has seizures is receiving physical therapy for a different condition, certain precautions must be made. High-pitched laser or extracorporeal shock wave treatment should be avoided, especially if used near the ears and head. Electrical stimulation should also be avoided near the head and neck, or used for short duration only and at low amplitude. Therapeutic exercise programs should be moderated so that dehydration or overexertion is avoided. Although regular exercise may be helpful in control of seizures, caution should be taken to minimize overstimulation.

A perfect clinical example to insert here is Guinness, a gorgeous five-year-old male English Mastiff, receiving physical therapy for hind limb weakness after cranial cruciate ligament surgery and a pinched nerve in the neck due to a bulged cervical spine disc. If this wasn't challenging enough, Guinness also suffered from idiopathic seizure disorder. Guinness' owners wisely chose chiropractic adjustments and active release treatment during the early acute phase of the disc problem, which helped to rapidly decrease the intensity of pain that had kept him from comfortably sitting and lying. After about nine days, physical therapy was initiated. Sub-acute pain, which radiated from his neck into the left forelimb needed to be addressed and the treatment of choice was laser and TENS. Due to the seizure risk, laser was used only on the lower portion of the neck, as far from the ears as possible with a cold pack placed about the spine to reduce inflammation and simultaneously help muffle the high-pitched signal produced by the laser. The TENS electrodes needed to be placed on the neck and along nerve pathways into the forelimb to control pain, but the pulse frequency and intensity were kept at the lowest levels possible. These modalities were used for very short durations to minimize risk of seizure inducement and massage, and joint mobilization and manual traction were applied immediately afterward. Guinness recovered quickly and no longer limped in pain on the left forelimb after two visits. Then we could begin to address the hind limb weakness and resume his daily leash walks to a nearby park. Guinness' owners knew that regular exercise was good for him in maintaining strength, endurance, and controlling body weight but they were always mindful to avoid extremes in temperature, humidity, and other weather conditions that might fatigue him and trigger seizure activity. Applying precautions and using a proactive approach during treatment is important when your animal has a seizure disorder.

Fibrocartilaginous Embolic Myelopathy (FCEM)

FCEM is a type of stroke that occurs in the spinal cord. It is caused by a tiny piece of fibrocartilage from the intervertebral disc, which forms a traveling body similar to a clot, in the blood vessels of the spine. It causes a lack of blood supply, occluding the blood vessels at a portion of the spinal cord, which produces neurological deficits. This can often be confused by pet owners with stroke or degenerative myelopathy, both of which differ from FCEM. A stroke occurs in the animal's brain, not the spinal cord. Degenerative myelopathy is non-inflammatory and occurs in the nerves through a stripping of the outer sheath. FCEM is an acute condition, displaying its effects right away, which appears suddenly during vigorous activity or trauma. It is not progressive, meaning that it does not worsen over time and usually displays the full extent of its damage within the first few hours. If it were a weather system, it would be more similar to a tornado than a slow-moving storm. Any region of the spinal cord can be affected with FCEM. When it occurs higher in the spinal cord, all four limbs are impaired. If it occurs in the middle or lower spinal cord, only the hind limbs will be impaired. It can produce signs on one or both sides of the animal's body. FCEM is not painful. Deficits can include weakness, paralysis, loss of coordination, abnormal motor tone, loss of sensation, etc. FCEM is diagnosed by ruling out other conditions such as disc disease, tumor, and arthritis along with tests like MRI, spinal tap, and myelogram.

FCEM tends to occur in large and giant breed dogs and in Miniature Schnauzers. It rarely occurs in small dogs, chondrodystrophic (dwarf) breeds like Dachshunds, or cats.

Spontaneous neurological recovery time is pretty quick with FCEM as most patients show their maximum recovery and improvement within the first twelve hours up to two weeks. Further improvement after this time is less likely to occur. Because of this, physical therapy should be started as early as possible, within a few hours to the first few days, unless the pet is medically unstable.

If the pet is unable to walk or move, your veterinarian will instruct you in nursing care, bowel and bladder management, nutrition, and other recommendations. The physical therapist will suggest the best padding and positioning, range of motion exercises for the limbs, and use of electrical stimulation (NMES) and massage to facilitate muscle activation. Slings and harnesses may be used to help the pet stand. Bolsters and Physio-Rolls or balls can support the pet for sitting and standing, with rolling and bouncing to help them begin to shift weight in preparation for walking. If knuckling or paw drop and dragging are present, a molded splint support can be helpful. Spinal joint mobilization and manipulation should not be performed on animals that have FCEM.

Vestibular and Balance Disorders

Nearly all of the conditions covered in this book affect an animal's ability to function through limits or restrictions in mobility. This section will describe conditions that pose the exact opposite problem: the presence of too much motion causing loss of control through the animal's body. Vestibular disorders cause ataxia, affecting balance and coordination of movement. There are four types of vestibular disorders:

1. Brain, affecting the cerebellum or brainstem caused by tumors, trauma, or vascular insults.
2. Spinal cord, also called "truncal ataxia," caused by trauma, compression of the dorsal part of the spinal cord carrying sensory messages to the brain.
3. Inner or middle ear, caused by infection, trauma, polyps, allergy, or congenital defect.
4. Idiopathic syndrome, affecting older geriatric animals, exact cause unknown.

The symptoms include head tilt to one side, stumbling and falling, staggering, incoordination, side-to-side eye movements (called "nystagmus"), and bumping into walls or objects. A trip to the veterinarian is needed for a complete diagnostic work-up and medical management before physical therapy is started. Infections and inflammation must be controlled first in order to prevent the condition from progressing. When the veterinarian feels the animal is stable, physical therapy can be initiated and will consist of various therapeutic exercises to address balance and coordination. The therapist will use various stimuli on the joints such as approximation (the opposite of traction), to facilitate muscles to co-contract and stabilize motion. Physio-Rolls and tilt boards can help restore balance. Small cuff weights may be attached to the animal's carpus (wrist) and hock (ankle) areas to slow down movement and help regain control of coordination. Manually guided techniques for rhythmical rocking back and forth, and from side to side, while the animal is standing up, can retrain motor planning ability. Various positionings of the head, neck, and body are used to reduce symptoms of inner and middle ear disturbances. Most of these exercises and techniques can be taught to the pet owner by a physical therapist to perform daily at home. There should be an emphasis on making good eye contact with your pet and using firm hand contact on its body during the exercises to provide sensory stimulation helpful for control of coordination and balance.

A lovely eight-year-old German Shorthaired Pointer named Abby suffered a sudden onset of ataxia with complete loss of ability to function one afternoon during an outdoor romp with her human dad. Although a definitive diagnosis was never fully determined, Abby's dad and veterinarian both knew that physical therapy would be important to maximize her potential to improve. On my initial visit to her home, she was lying on a blanket, only able to raise her head and unable to control the movements necessary to stand or walk. Being a sporting dog, she was desperate to be active and through sheer determination, moved about the room by sliding on her side. Heartbreaking indeed! However, the story has a happy ending that is a testament to three factors: Abby's strong will, her dad's positive and loving attitude, and early initiation of physical therapy. Utilizing many of the physical therapy treatment techniques addressed above and her dad using his carpentry skills to build a standing scaffold with slings and harness, Abby soared through the recovery process. Within a month, she was able to walk on her own, exploring the woods and climbing over stones and branches. She has some residual weakness of one forelimb and a few balance deficits, but can function well under the loving supervision of her dad.

Neuromuscular Disease

These diseases are somewhat rare but quite disabling and problematic. Neuromuscular symptoms develop when disease or infection attacks and damages the signal connection between the nerves and muscles. This neuromuscular junction is a physical gap present at every motor point in the body, where the nerves enter a muscle. When the nerve is signaled to stimulate a muscle contraction, it releases chemical messengers, called "neurotransmitters," to bridge the gap. These transmitters communicate with receptor sites in muscles, which complete the action necessary for it to contract. When this process is impaired, it results in weakness, muscle tremors, stiffness, clumsy walking, and even problems with swallowing and breathing. It can be seen in dogs as well as cats and is diagnosed through blood work, radiographs, spinal tap, and electromyography. The condition can be inherited or acquired through toxins, in addition to the causes mentioned above.

Physical therapy is very important in the treatment and management of animals with neuromuscular disease. Muscles that are tight need to be carefully stretched in a manner that does not exacerbate the excitability of nerves. If the limb is not handled correctly, pressure on certain locations of the paw may set off clonus, a reflexive shaking or beating movement of the paw. Therefore, the therapist must be knowledgeable in correct hand placement and technique to release the tightness, while maintaining relaxed muscle tone. There are strengthening exercises that can help to maintain functional tone and use of muscles, but they rarely improve the condition. Physical therapy is also helpful in the dog's walking and balance. Bracing of the hind limbs is often helpful and the therapist or veterinarian can assist with recommendation of lightweight products.

A gentle giant named Rocky entered my life as a patient about two years ago. Rocky is now a ten-year-old Newfoundland that has a devoted and loving family anxious to help him function with his unfortunate diagnosis of neuromuscular disease. To make matters more challenging, Rocky also has cranial cruciate ligament tears. Several veterinary surgeons evaluated Rocky and the final outcome was to do conservative treatment instead of surgery, due to the neuromuscular disease and its likelihood to affect his strength. Physical therapy, medications, and supplements became very important to Rocky and still help him to this day! Rocky has tight, spastic muscles and walks slowly with some rotation of a hind limb, but he has been able to meet all of his physical therapy goals and maintain them with monthly in-home visits of laser, massage, stretching, and Thera Band resistive strengthening. He no longer drags his limbs as severely or labors to stand up and can take short leash walks in the neighborhood, greeting his human friends, and keeping up with his social activities!

Toxicity

Along with neuromuscular disease, toxic exposure can cause a variety of disorders in animals. One example is tetanus, which occurs when a dog is infected with the clostridium tetani bacteria. These bacteria, often found outdoors in soil and manure, infect the animal through deep cuts or puncture wounds. Once infected, the bacteria release toxins that bind to nerves. In serious cases, toxins are transported along the outer peripheral nerve pathways until reaching the central nervous system, where it is usually fatal. In milder cases, it does not reach the central nervous system and is called "focal tetanus." I worked with a darling Boston Terrier, Kava, who had focal tetanus affecting one of his front limbs. He required extensive therapy to relax abnormal muscle tone and restore the maximum range of motion in the shoulder. With tetanus, toxins block the normal inhibitory mechanisms that control muscle excitability, resulting in hard spasms and rigid muscle tone. The affected muscles stay in a prolonged contracted state, resulting in pain and disability. Muscle relaxants and sedatives are normally prescribed to relieve symptoms. Physical therapy can be helpful in relieving muscle tone and increasing range of motion. Specific manual techniques are used along with massage, stretching, propping the dog over bolsters or rolls, and using laser over areas of joint tightness. Special molded splints that help inhibit the excitability of nerves can be fabricated by the therapist or a specialist who makes braces.

The prognosis for tetanus varies greatly. I have seen dogs and cats that improve with physical therapy and medication, and others that result in limb amputation when conservative treatment is unsuccessful. The Boston Terrier Kava did well with physical therapy for a few months until his muscle tone took an unexpected and dramatic turn, becoming much worse and requiring limb amputation. He remains a happy and fun-loving dog, chasing down every tennis ball thrown his way!

Lockjaw can be caused by a tetanus infection. The affected muscles here are the chewing muscles in the cheek (masseter) and muscles on the sides of the head that help in closing the mouth (temporalis). Other causes can be muscle inflammation, severe arthritis, and abnormal bone growth in the jaw region.

I had a very challenging case involving a pretty, nine-year-old Shar Pei, Jasmine, who was unable to open her mouth. The initial diagnosis was lock jaw from tetanus, until the final blood work results revealed a different cause. The veterinarian explained to me that there is a special antibody test using blood and muscle tissue samples that can diagnose an inflammatory condition called myositis. Jasmine, it turned out, had masticatory myositis, an inflammation of the masseter muscle. She was unable to open her mouth and had to be fed with liquids and broth using a plastic syringe pried between her teeth. Jasmine was losing weight and the veterinarian was highly concerned that the condition would soon become life threatening. High doses of prednisone were given to Jasmine to relieve this inflammation but the results were slow and the veterinarian began to search other ways to help Jasmine. A colleague of this doctor suggested physical therapy and I received an urgent call to start treatment. I had never treated an animal with this condition and was unsure what to expect. Jasmine presented with hollow cheeks, due to atrophy and shrinkage of the muscle fibers in the cheek, not from lack of nutrition. These muscles, the masseters, felt hard and tender when touched both on the outside of the face and internally from inside the mouth at the cheek lining. She was unable to open her mouth due to the resistance of inflamed and tight chewing muscles, but it could be passively pried open using my hands, approximately one-quarter of an inch. I started physical therapy immediately using moist hot packs and laser over the jaw (TMJ) joint and masseter muscles of the cheek. I also applied TENS (electrical stimulation) for pain relief, massage, and joint gliding techniques for the jaw. I discussed possible ways to stretch the jaw safely with the veterinarian. In my human physical therapy experience, a thin stack of wood tongue depressors would be used, placed between the teeth to provide a slow, steady stretch. However, this would not be safe for an animal if the force of its teeth cracked the wood and splinters were swallowed, etc. We decided to use small strips of rawhide chews, dipped in canned dog food, to place between her teeth in thirty to sixty second intervals. Gradually, over the next few days, Jasmine's jaw began to relax slightly. The hospital staff began to feed her diluted canned dog food, which she was able to drink now that her tongue could emerge. Within two weeks, Jasmine was able to bark and lick her lips. The canned food no longer needed diluting to the point of liquid, but to that of thick batter. Her mouth now opened to one-half an inch. Over the next few weeks, Jasmine's cheeks were less hollow as the muscles started to relax and expand. She began to eat small puppy-sized kibble and mini dog treats, with her mouth opening one inch. At this point, the veterinarian began to taper the prednisone dosage. Gradual medication weaning and steady physical therapy treatment over the course of six months resulted in Jasmine being able to open her mouth approximately three inches and eat a full normal diet of wet and dry food, with treats. She eventually was fully weaned off the prednisone and physical therapy was discontinued. Although she was never able to open her mouth fully, the results gave her a satisfactory and functional range of motion.

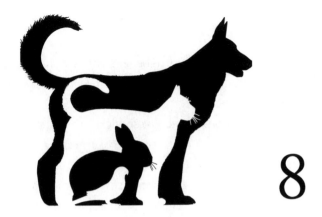

8

Rehabilitation of Medical Conditions

Oncology

There may be no category of veterinary illness that causes greater angst and heartbreak for the pet owner than that of oncology (cancer). Helplessness and desperation are the emotions I often hear when contacted by prospective clients whose pets are undergoing treatment for cancer. The need to do something is foremost in his or her mind. Until recently, physical therapy was not associated with treatments to help cancer patients, but human medicine is now utilizing it most effectively. The same principles of physical therapy that are helping people with cancer hold true for animals!

The primary treatments for cancer patients are surgery, chemotherapy, and radiation therapy. The effects of cancer treatments can be quite debilitating and include pain, fatigue, weakness, low endurance, decreased ability to function, and impaired walking. Using appropriate physical therapy interventions to combat these side effects gives comfort to both the pet and its owner. The results can be seen with improved quality of life, maintaining the ability to function, lessened risk of injury, and stress management.

Specifically, physical therapy services can be utilized to assist in the recovery from cancer-related surgery as well as helping the body respond to the assaults of chemo and radiation treatments. All of these cancer treatments require some level of physical strength and endurance, before and after they are administered. Emerging evidence in human medicine suggests that exercise and conditioning can increase physiological and even psychological functioning, which help to maximize the therapeutic effects of cancer treatment.

Examples of physical therapy interventions used in the treatment of animal patients having cancer include massage over sore and tight muscles, lymphatic massage techniques to manage swelling of the limbs, friction massage over surgery incisions, joint range of motion, positioning for comfort and support, and therapeutic exercises. What you will *not* see in the physical therapy treatment of cancer patients is the use of physical modalities such as laser and ultrasound as they are contraindicated. Laser and ultrasound are deep in penetration and serve to increase cellular permeability and metabolism, which could cause a dangerous proliferation of cancer cells.

Therapeutic exercise reduces the intensity of cancer treatment-related fatigue. The program of exercise designed by the therapist should be gentle, comfortable, and graded. Exercise intensity should be submaximal, with a gradual progression of its duration. The activities given to perform will be structured and consistent, without the use of interval bursts. Interval training, helpful in sports, agility, and weight management are not appropriate here. Slow and steady should be the mantra during the course of physical therapy exercises in cancer rehabilitation. The following is an example of an exercise program typical for use during cancer treatment:

Five to six reps of push-pull extremity exercise, using gentle manual resistance or light yellow or red Thera Bands, followed by a five second rest, repeated three to four times.

Sit to stand three times, followed by walking across the room, turning, and walking back. Rest thirty seconds. Repeat four times.

Standing on a mat or carpet, using toys or treats to cue the pet to look up, down, and side to side for one to two minutes.

Standing on mat or carpet, raise one front limb up several inches and hold three seconds. Repeat four times. Perform the same on other front limb. Progress to lifting the rear limbs, one at a time. If the animal cannot tolerate this or is unable to maintain its balance, place the limb on a low surface such as a book or piece of wood approximately one to two inches in vertical height, and help hold its body steady for five to ten seconds.

Take slow leash walks of ten to twelve minutes, one to two times per day, on level surfaces. Gradually progress to adding some low-rise slopes or inclines.

Place two chairs about eight feet apart (for a medium-sized dog) and use a leash to guide the pet walking around the chairs in a figure-eight pattern, three times. Then reverse the direction for three repetitions.

These are samples of many types of activities or exercises that a therapist might carefully select for your pet. The actual parameters vary depending on the pet's size and level of conditioning, and are gradually progressed as tolerated. You will be asked to record your pet's current levels of activity, movement, rest, eating, and bowel/bladder habits, and keep a daily diary. This will be reviewed every one to two weeks to assess the pet's tolerance and progress. It is a helpful tool to track the effectiveness of your efforts and you will likely be very encouraged by the results!

Physical therapy should not be given if an infection is present or if the animal is experiencing cardiovascular or respiratory impairments. The veterinarian can advise when it is safe to resume treatment.

I'd like to share the stories of two very different oncology canine cases I was involved with:

First is Lincoln, a nine-year-old male Chocolate Lab, with a history of two cranial cruciate ligament surgical repairs and degenerative arthritis of the spine. He received physical rehabilitation for his orthopedic problems and did well for two years. When his family began to notice that Lincoln was having difficulty getting up from the floor, less control of the hind limbs, frequent bowel accidents, weight loss, and low appetite, they took him to the veterinarian. After several tests, Lincoln was diagnosed with multiple myeloma, a malignancy seen in larger breed dogs, with a large extradural tumor on his spine. The condition was quite advanced and treatment options were limited. The family opted to decline chemotherapy and focus on quality of life care for his remaining time. I was contacted to evaluate Lincoln and formulate an appropriate treatment plan. Lincoln was anxious and fearful when I initially met him.

He was very unstable with walking and often slipped and fell in the house. He still had some sparkle in his eyes and seemed to enjoy being with the family and other household pets. My overall goal for physical therapy was supportive and focused on maximizing his ease of functioning and providing comfort. I utilized massage of the limbs, in particular the forelimbs, which displayed swelling in the paws. This was a lymphatic drainage type of massage technique, performed with Lincoln lying on his side, with the limb elevated on a beanbag. Range of motion to the joints with light stretching of his hamstrings and Achilles tendons was next, which helped him relax. A 53-cm peanut-shaped Physio-Roll was used to support Lincoln in the standing position, with maximal assistance from me and one family member to lift and guide him over it. This allowed his spine to elongate and de-load his elbows and stifle joints. I used a sling assist looped under his belly to aide walking down the back door steps and out into the yard. Several modifications were suggested to help Lincoln function better indoors, such as the use of elevated food and water bowls, placement of non-skid mats and carpet runners over wood and tile floors to prevent slips, and positioning Lincoln's bed on an elevated palette for ease of getting in and rising from it. Traction boots, incontinence garments, and a lifting harness were also recommended (see Appendix: Helpful Resources). To help preserve strength, Lincoln was transported to a local canine pool facility, which allowed buoyant support for his arthritic joints while he used his muscles to swim, aided by a floatation jacket with ropes. This was a great mood elevator, for this water-loving Lab.

Sadly, Lincoln lost his battle and was peacefully euthanized about six weeks later, but his family felt satisfaction that his last few weeks were comfortable and happy ones. I was grateful to have the opportunity to play a helpful role in his final few weeks of earthly life.

Next is Merlot, an eleven-year-old Weimaraner who shares his home with his human mom and two other dogs of the same breed. Merlot has had two surgeries to remove malignant tumors in the spinal and ribcage regions. These were spindle cell sarcomas that were large and oval-shaped, easily seen and felt. With the first surgery, Merlot had accompanying lameness in his right hind limb. The surgeon felt this could have been the result of a small stroke (Merlot also has a history of high blood pressure) or an inflamed spinal nerve root caused by swelling or scar tissue. After the second surgery, a period of chemotherapy was administered, resulting in fatigue with lethargy and weakness. Merlot was regularly attending canine swim along with in-home Reiki sessions. Both were quite helpful yet he still lacked control of the hind limb, limped, and had frequent episodes of falling. Physical therapy was recommended and Merlot was evaluated in his home. Goals were set for improving his gait pattern, which displayed scissoring and knuckling at the right hind limb, achieving better control on the stairs, reducing or eliminating falls, and increasing strength and energy level. Laser was applied to his elbows, but I avoided using it along the spine where the tumors were removed, even though the surgeon reported clean margins post-operatively. Cross-friction massage and myofascial release were performed over the incisions to reduce scarring and adherence of connective tissue to the ribcage. Range of motion and stretching were applied to tightness at the right hip and hock (ankle). Functional stimulation electrodes were placed on the foot elevator muscles at the outer shin and on the thigh quadriceps to build tone and bulk.

Strengthening exercises using a medium red Thera Band and a sand-filled cuff weight were performed in the side lying and standing positions. Additional balance and strength activities using a Physio-Roll, balance bubble, and walk-around cones were included in treatment. Merlot's walking began to improve with more control of the right hind limb, especially on carpeted surfaces, on outdoor grass, and pavement. His falls were not eliminated but greatly reduced in number. Merlot became less reluctant to use the stairs and had greater control, especially when ascending. He required supervision when descending as this activity utilizes eccentric or controlled lengthening contractions of the hip/thigh muscles. Leash walks were encouraged, interspersed with short intervals of faster speed and trotting. Merlot's large backyard offered sloped inclines that he could climb up and down to further increase his strength.

Merlot continues to do well and receives maintenance PT every two weeks. His mom reports that Merlot is brighter and more energetic after each therapy session. He has been able to achieve increased bulk, measured in circumference of the thigh, and strength rated as good minus at the right hind limb. He usually runs to greet me when I ring the doorbell, no longer slipping or struggling!

Amputation

The thought of a missing limb is not at all pleasant to consider, but animals cope with it quite well. Limb amputation is a surgical procedure to remove a limb due to disease or injury. The indications to have a limb amputated are pain, dangerous tumors such as osteosarcoma (bone cancer) or soft tissue sarcoma, severe trauma with multiple fractures, injury to the blood supply of the limb, birth defects, etc. In some trauma or birth defect cases, physical therapy can be utilized successfully to save a limb, but in cases where there is no rehabilitation potential, amputation is the best option. Animals are extremely adaptable and most do well as a tripod during play, walking, and running. They are accustomed to walking on four points of contact with the ground, compared to two in a human, so that the loss of one limb is not distressing. The animal limb is not designed for fine motor skills as a human's, so this factor also lessens the impact of limb loss to animal. Amputation is far worse for the human owner!

Front limb amputation can be slightly more difficult than rear limb, as normal body weight distribution is shifted forward in animals, mostly due to the weight of the head and neck. Approximately 60 percent of body weight is borne on the front limbs and 40 percent on the rear.

Physical therapy can be very beneficial after limb amputation for wound care and use of laser to facilitate quick healing. Incision mobilization and massage techniques can help prevent and breakdown scar tissue. Manually handling and lightly rubbing the skin surface by the incision can help desensitize and prevent phantom limb pain (or phantom limb sensation). Stretching needs to be done for muscles that become tight as the pet may try to tuck the residual portion of its remaining limb under the body initially. Assistance with balance and weight shifting is helpful in the early days after surgery to help the pet quickly adjust to the redistribution due to loss of limb.

The physical therapist can be most helpful in suggesting the following assistive devices, environmental modifications, and mobility aides or prosthetic devices:

1. A standing and walking harness placed under the chest for front limb amputees, or a sling placed under the belly for hind limb amputees
2. Non-slip carpets, runners, or mats in strategic locations in the home
3. Low-rise ramps for getting in/out of the house
4. Shallow litter pans for feline amputees
5. Wheeled carts for pets that have difficulty moving and walking as a tripod
6. Prosthetic (artificial limb) recommendations

While many dogs and cats manage beautifully as tripods, others may have a more difficult time due to age; being overweight; having arthritis or dysplasia in other joints; the presence of a neurological, cardiac, or respiratory condition, etc. In these cases, prosthesis can be considered. The best candidates are those pets whose amputation is farther down on the limb. This provides a stump, leaving adequate room to attach a prosthesis. The prosthesis consists of a false limb with an open socket and suspension system: the socket is slipped over the stump and secured with suspension straps. The simplest and easiest prosthesis to use is below the knee or below the elbow amputees. Animals that have amputations above the knee or elbow usually have a shorter stump from which to attach the prostheses, need bulky suspension harnesses, and require the device to have an artificial joint. These prostheses are more complex and expensive, with hydraulic piston joints. Many times a wheeled cart is more practical in these types of amputations.

New advances in animal prosthetics include osseointegration, in which the device is connected to living tissue and bone. It is similar to dentistry with artificial tooth implants. This technique uses a titanium alloy anchor made of carbon fiber or composite material that is screwed into bone and fitted onto the prosthesis. Then, bone and skin literally grow around it over time. This is rapidly becoming the future of animal prosthetics.

Prosthetic devices aren't just for dogs and cats: they are commonly used as bird beaks, fish fins, turtle feet, and with elephants and horses!

(See Note 16.)

Metabolic Diseases

Metabolic diseases arise from the disruption of organs and their cells to function optimally and together with other organs in the body. Examples of these conditions are Cushing's, diabetes, anemia, etc. You may not associate these diseases with the need for physical therapy treatment, but therapists have been helping human patients afflicted with metabolic disorders for many years. This has carried over into the veterinary profession as doctors and technicians working with animals are realizing the vast benefits of PT.

Cushing's disease is a hormonal hyper-imbalance of the adrenal gland where too much cortisol is produced. This hyper adrenal corticism causes skin problems, bloat and abdominal distention, increased appetite with weight gain, muscle weakness, and suppressed immune system. This condition is much more common in animals than its mirror image, Addison's disease. A physical therapist can play an important role in helping an animal with Cushing's by recognizing any signs of early infection, which are masked by immunosuppression, and refer to a veterinarian for medical follow-up. Physical therapy is also helpful to establish exercise programs to help increase muscle strength, avoid weight gain, and improve bone mass as well as endurance levels.

With Addison's disease, a physical therapist assumes a completely different approach. This condition is characterized by adrenal insufficiency, or hypoadrenocorticism. An animal usually has low appetite, a dull countenance, low energy level, and gastrointestinal disturbances. Whereas physical therapists need to push their Cushing's patients into effort and activity, the "no pain, no gain" method works poorly with Addison's disease. A more passive approach to therapy is indicated, with structured rest periods, avoidance of external heat and humidity, and emphasis on the maintenance of joint range of motion rather than on muscle strengthening.

Diabetes in animals is another metabolic condition in which physical therapy plays an important role. Due to circulatory disturbances, wounds and their healing are problematic. Treatment with whirlpool, irrigation, medicated dressings, and the use of laser can be used by the physical therapist to help with wound healing. If neuropathy occurs, along with decreased sensation, the therapist can coach the pet owner in avoiding obstacles that can cause slipping and other injury. A splint or brace might be needed to support the paw and hock/ankle joint in cases of dropped foot. Exercise programs, primarily the aerobic type, can be designed to help metabolize glucose, in the absence of insulin produced by the pancreas.

Imbalance of thyroid hormone can also cause conditions that may benefit from physical therapy. Hyperthyroidism in cats can cause muscle weakness, requiring general conditioning and strengthening exercises. Hypothyroidism in dogs can create various myotonias, or abnormal motor tone, requiring stretching and muscular relaxation techniques.

Rickets is a bone disorder, characterized by loss of mineralization, similar to osteopenia. There is also disruption of the formation and functioning of the bony growth plates. It is caused by inadequate dietary calcium and vitamins during early stages of life. The animal often presents with stunted growth, curvature in the long bones, deformity at various joints, and muscle weakness. Physical therapy can be beneficial in providing range of motion exercises, muscle strengthening, graded weight bearing, aerobic exercise programs, and consultation regarding splints or braces and mobility devices. All of the rickets cases that have been referred to me over the years have been essentially caused by neglect with poor nutrition and some type of movement restriction with cage or crate confinement. These cases are very difficult.

There are other types of metabolic disturbances, besides rickets, that can be caused by neglect and abuse. One such case is a famous Pit Bull named Patrick, who was found starved and abandoned in Newark, New Jersey. Poor Patrick, near death, suffered dehydration, hypothermia, muscle wasting, dangerous electrolyte levels, and stress to the liver and other organs, etc.

Here is a description of the type of physical therapy treatment needed to help Patrick and other animals that have survived starvation and neglect:

Therapy was provided twice per week for two months. After assessing Patrick's deficits and setting rehabilitation goals, I knew my treatment approach would need to be modified, due to the effects of prolonged starvation and neglect. Patrick was very debilitated and had decreased muscle mass. There was tightness in the tendons of his left hind limb, likely due to his positioning while lying and being too weak to move. The hospital staff noted that Patrick favored this limb, especially in the morning upon waking. Thus, there was potential for his treatment to injure him if not done with considerable care. I had to balance providing enough therapy each session to obtain results without being overly aggressive, in order to avoid soreness and strain.

Therapy began with a soothing type of massage called "effleurage," Reiki, range of motion, and stretching tight hind limb muscles and tendons. Techniques were gentle, slow, and performed only a few repetitions at a time. I usually held Patrick and draped him across my lap for this phase of care. He was so sweet and cooperative. I would lift Patrick and help him to stand to support weight evenly on all four limbs, using an inflated Physio-Roll, rocker board, and balance bubble.

Soon Patrick regained full range of motion and stopped favoring the left hind limb. His coat became thicker, his energy level increased, and he started taking short leash walks outdoors. PT treatment then began to focus on building muscle mass and strength, by using functional exercises which were fun for Patrick, used the whole body, and were highly efficient to conserve his energy. Strengthening also included the abdominal and spine, or "core" groups. Patrick began to take longer walks, climbing steps, walking up/down inclines, around trees, on varying surfaces, and enjoying interactive play with toys. Mini intervals of increased speed or intensity would be inserted, to further ramp up his endurance, similar to sprint intervals done by runners. Patrick soared through his PT and seemed to enjoy every moment, gaining steady improvement each week. He now stood with even weight distribution, normal top line, increased speed with walking, more muscle bulk, and less fatigue. In addition to PT, he received ongoing expert medical care by the hospital and sessions by a distance Reiki healer.

Geriatrics

Advances in veterinary medicine over the past fifteen or more years have done much to improve and lengthen an animal's life span. The same is true for human counterparts who are living longer and more active lives. Increased medical awareness of the effects of human aging is evident with the emergence of specialty physicians called gerontologists. I predict that the veterinary field will produce such specialists, including specialty rehabilitation and physical therapists to address unique issues affecting older animals.

Your veterinarian is usually the best person to determine when your pet is entering its senior years. It is based on size, breed, and other factors in addition to chronological age. Obviously, a seven-year-old Mastiff and a seven-year-old Dachshund would both not be considered geriatric. The veterinarian can also advise you on the best supplements and nutrition for your pet at this stage of its life. Some changes might include decreasing the intake or amount of food, changing the texture or consistency, adding more protein, and choosing food that incorporates certain vitamins and minerals.

Your physical therapist may be the best person to guide you in terms of activity, exercise, and lifestyle. In my practice, I focus on three main areas with my geriatric animal patients:

1. Quality of daily life: Physical and mental stimulation are important ingredients to helping a geriatric pet maintain enjoyment in its life. Simple range of motion exercises done in the morning can ease stiff joints after sleep. Because older pets tend to sleep more, and move about slower, their joints are subject to loss

of general mobility (not to be confused with arthritis) as they age. You might need to spend more time touching and stroking your pet, along with talking or singing to it as it can lose tactile sensation, sight, and hearing. This added one-on-one time can provide good stimulation to help them retain and sharpen its available senses. You should approach a sight- or hearing-impaired animal slowly and carefully, and keep its environment consistent in the placement of its bed, toys, and food. Provide familiar sounds and smells to help guide the animal in direction and location. Cats may need assistance with brushing and cleaning, as they tend to lose their ability to perform self-grooming as they age. There are mental changes that also appear with some pets as they become older such as anxiety, depression, and even dementia. You may notice a cat or dog being more vocal or pacing around, not being able to get comfortable. In these situations, it is best to confine it to a smaller area, where it has fewer choices to make, but choose an area where things are going on, such as the kitchen or den. Let the pet watch you cook, work on crafts or projects, and keep music or a television on in the background. Most of all, smile and say a cheerful word to it often!

2. Ability to function safely: At this stage of their life, animals need modifications and some proactive planning by their owner or family, to ensure safety and avoid injury. An older pet's muscle tone begins to decrease, its cardiac output may be reduced, metabolism slows, bones and nails might tend to be brittle,

and the immune system may not be as competent. You will need to look over your home or the pet's environment with a critical eye and make adaptations needed for negotiating stairs, climbing on/off a couch, jumping up to a cat condo landing, balancing and holding onto roosting posts, etc. Ramps should be built, with side walls and non-skid runners. Beds may need extra padding or elevation to make climbing into and out of easier. Food and water dishes or troughs may need a change in height. Your cat may need a different kind of litter box if it has difficulty entering and exiting. Feline condos or climbing poles may need to be modified and platforms lowered. Older dogs tend to need more frequent potty breaks as they may urinate more often. Exercise remains very important for seniors as staying active helps curb some of the negative effects of aging. The difference is in the discernment of what type of exercise or walking environment may pose risks for your pet. For example, if your dog loves walks but has a lowered immune system, you should choose city or sidewalk walking over the forest, woods, or grassy fields. During the walks, you need to stay off cell phones and tablets and look ahead for potholes, glass, or ice that your older dog might not see, or scraps of tempting food that could be hazardous. I recommend shorter, more frequent leash walks and at consistent times, whenever possible. Although animals always enjoy variety, they need more structure and consistency as they age. Exercise should be easily tolerated and of low impact: avoiding hard climbing, jumping, uneven terrain, or heavy play with other pets. If strengthening is needed, a physical therapist can guide you in an appropriate home program that may contain more open chain movements done in lying down or sitting positions and less emphasis on functional exercises.

3. Having a purpose: It is important to keep older animals active and engaged in purposeful life activity. They like to have a job to do and one of their favorite jobs is looking after the family. The value of this was taught to me by a group of goats I had the pleasure of working with. One of the advantages of being a mobile, on-site physical therapist for animals is the variety of places I visit on my patient care rounds. I've been to the New Jersey Pinelands, the floating houses of Margate near Atlantic City, the cities of Newark and Elizabeth, and the mountains in northwestern New Jersey, along with zoos and farms.

In 2009, I was asked to visit a farm to evaluate a rescued geriatric goat named Lucia. Lucia had been neglected and her hooves were grossly overgrown, causing her to stand and walk on the front wrist (carpus) joints, with her forelimbs bent and buckled underneath her. Normally, a goat in the wild will automatically self-trim its hooves by climbing on the mountain terrain or steppes. Dairy goats' hooves have to be hand trimmed and if allowed to overgrow, can cripple a goat, as Lucia.

Now in a safe facility, her guardian engaged the services of a local veterinarian and farrier to tackle the laborious job of hoof trimming done with a dremel over several tedious hours. After the hooves were trimmed to their proper length and balanced, the physical therapy evaluation could commence. I found poor Lucia's tendons to have contracted and shortened, preventing her from being able to stand fully upright, even though she now had normal hoof length. My job was clear: range of motion must be restored, along with reduction of the contracture so that Lucia could return to a full life of standing to forage in the grass and play with new friends. The physical therapy treatment consisted of gentle massage, stretching the tight tendons, and range of motion to the joints of the forelimb. As the tightness reduced and her joints loosened, I assisted her to fully standing with her weight on the extended forelimbs, while supporting her under the chest. We would rock slowly back and forth and side to side in weight-shifting exercises, which gradually gave her confidence and strength to stand fully upright. Over the course of three months, Lucia gained full range of motion, strength, and the ability to stand, walk, and function fairly normally as a goat. Occasionally, she was seen in her prior downward propped position, but this was attributed to habit or fatigue.

I was recalled a few weeks later to check Lucia again since she was favoring her former buckled stand position more and more. Her range of motion remained normal, the contractures absent, and her hooves regularly maintained. There was no apparent physical reason for Lucia to resume the prior postures when her hooves were overgrown. Was it simply habit? There was nothing more I could offer Lucia in terms of physical therapy.

Enter two baby goats, or kids, rescued and brought to the same facility where elderly Lucia now lived. These little darlings, homeless and injured, also needed physical therapy for weakness after a virus. They were splendid PT patients with full recovery and ready to be transferred to a permanent farm home, though none had yet been found. In the meantime, Lucia's guardian, having no other space to put the kids, decided to house them temporarily with Lucia. Can you figure out the end of this story? At first, Lucia ignored the kids, but within days, she no longer stood crumpled on her front legs, but fully upright with her front hooves and carpus joints extended with head high! Of course—the problem was more than physical all along! After the physical issues were resolved, she needed a job and a purpose! The two kids are no longer homeless and have a new adopted mom in Lucia, and Lucia is proud and busy helping raise the two young charges. No out-placements are needed as this family will stay together and help each other. Anyone reading this who is adopted (as I am) or has adopted a child knows that parenthood has more to do with who raises you than with genetics. Lucia and her two kids demonstrate this beautifully along with the importance of having duty and purpose in your life. My frequent visits to Lucia and her brood are no longer for PT but to praise her, admire the (now) yearlings, and experience the joyous lessons they have taught me!

Arthritis

There are three basic types of arthritis seen in animals: the most common being osteoarthritis (OA), also called "degenerative joint disease" (DJD). The other two forms are autoimmune and systemic, similar to rheumatoid arthritis in human beings and infectious arthritis, caused by an organism entering a joint and becoming septic.

I will focus on osteoarthritis, as it is prevalent and commonly treated with physical therapy. There are two forms of OA: primary, or idiopathic (unknown cause), seen in older animals, overweight animals, and in certain breeds; and secondary, resulting from a prior condition such as dysplasia, trauma, congenital joint defects, etc. Both types are characterized by wear and tear on weight-bearing joints, with inflammation, stiffness, and pain. The part of the joint most affected by arthritis is the articular cartilage. Articular cartilage covers the ends of long bones and acts like a waterbed for an animal's weight-bearing joints. It distributes forces during contact stress from loads produced during standing, walking, running, playing, etc. This cartilage does not have a blood supply, lymph nodes, or nerve endings. However, when it becomes eroded or damaged, the result is pain and inflammation, due to grinding, bone touching bone, and inflammation of the surrounding joint capsule and synovial (lubricating) fluid.

Arthritis is diagnosed by radiographs and examination. Animals with OA typically stand with a rounded topline, especially toward the rear end, with the hind limbs tucked underneath the body. They tend to sit with the hind limbs extended straight out, instead of having the knees bent. Range of motion is usually decreased, and a crackling sound or grinding feel, called "crepitus," is present.

Arthritis is best treated with a multi-modal approach, combining medications, supplements, weight management, acupuncture, and physical therapy. Physical therapy modalities such as heat applications, continuous ultrasound, laser, TENS, and massage are often very helpful. These modalities take on even greater importance when an animal is unable to take various medications such as NSAIDS to control pain. Therapeutic exercise is also critical for arthritis management. Studies show that static stress leads more to the erosion of articular cartilage than intermittent stress. This finding tells us that body movement as well as range of motion of individual joints is beneficial for arthritic animals. However, this movement needs to be controlled, mild in intensity, and of low impact. Examples of this are exercises over a Physio-Roll or Thera Ball, swimming, underwater treadmill walking, active-assisted range of motion, gentle stretching, and Grade 1 and 2 joint mobilizations, etc. Types of exercises that should be avoided are joint manipulations, use of heavy resistance bands or weights, agility, heavy play with other pets, excessive trotting, intervals, and jumping. Harnesses, slings, and other supports for the elbows, hips, shoulders, and spine can be used during activity, especially in cold, damp weather. Arthritic pets should have soft, padded beds, blankets or other means of providing heat, and carpet or non-skid flooring. Some animals may prefer to lie down on cooler surfaces such as tile or cement floors at times of acute inflammation of their joints, but they may need assistance in rising. Leash walks are great forms of exercise for arthritic animals, but they should be shorter and more frequent, spaced evenly throughout the day: three walks, ten to fifteen minutes each.

If your veterinarian has prescribed supplements for your pet, they can be taken in tandem with physical therapy treatments, without interruption. The same holds true for anti-inflammatory medications, if they are prescribed in therapeutic doses. If these medications are prescribed on an as-needed basis, they should be stopped at least six hours prior to physical therapy treatment, so that pain is not masked and the therapist can judge your pet's tolerance. Medication can be administered right after the therapy session is over. Cold packs can also be applied at that time, to reduce any inflammation. (See Note 17.)

I have seen many patients having chronic osteoarthritis benefit from conservative management and physical therapy. Two memorable cases are:

1. Teddy, a darling thirteen-year-old mini lop-eared house rabbit, diagnosed with osteoarthritis (OA) of his hips and elbows. Teddy had nearly lost all mobility, barely being able to hop. When he did, he struggled painfully and slowly, dragging his right rear limb. In sitting, Teddy held his right rear limb out to the side and rotated inwardly. He also stopped grooming his face with his front paws, as he was too uncomfortable to sit on the hind limbs alone, and needed to use his front limbs for support. Teddy's mom Robin was beginning to think that Teddy would need to be put down if they couldn't find a solution since the anti-inflammatory medication was not helping sufficiently. Robin was having her own problems with a painful arthritic condition of her spine and had just started physical therapy. She asked her veterinarian if PT might help Teddy and soon after that, I was contacted to evaluate and provide treatment. Little Teddy was a terrific patient and did well with his treatment, consisting of a warm towel body wrap, gentle massage, range of motion exercises, and stretching over a roll. Well, not a typical Physio-Roll, but a homemade roll made out of a round oatmeal container, sized perfectly for a small rabbit. After about five weeks, Teddy

was hopping with greater ease, less dragging of the rear limb, sitting up for longer periods, and able to resume some grooming activity!

2. Othello is a handsome fourteen-year-old domestic short-haired cat with degenerative arthritis of the right hip. He gradually became unable to jump up onto his favorite look-out perches and walked with a stiff, guarded gait, holding the right hind limb stiffly. Radiographs were taken, confirming the OA, and physical therapy ordered. Othello received laser treatments, massage, range of motion, joint mobilization techniques to the hip, stretching to the hip and thigh musculature, and gentle weight shifting with rocking, standing on a balance bubble. I also placed him over my shoulder, while providing a gentle traction stretch to his hip, which seemed to be his favorite part of the session (probably because I threw a few good hugs in!). Othello still walked with a slight limp, but began to resume jumping and climbing (albeit slowly and carefully) on his kitty tree once again.

Respiratory Illness

An animal patient's respiratory system can be affected by various conditions such as rib fractures; injury to the head, neck, or chest; abdominal or thoracic surgery; or any critical illness requiring prolonged rest. As a result, the animal may be unable to cough effectively or breathe as deeply, and lung congestion and other respiratory complications may develop. Physical therapists use the techniques of postural drainage positioning, manual percussion, and vibration to treat these conditions in humans and animals. I've had several occasions to use these techniques in animals such as Deary, a young goat with an injury to the ribcage, and Guinness, an English Mastiff that had abdominal surgery to remove carpet fragments that he had ingested.

Postural drainage involves positioning the animal on its back, stomach, and side, with wedges and pillows to allow gravity to drain secretions and congestion from various parts of the lung. Lungs are divided into different segments, and the therapist will use specific positions to drain the parts of the lung most affected. Determining which lung segments are affected is done by chest X-ray and listening to breathing patterns with a stethoscope.

After a few minutes of this positioning, the therapist will cup her hands with fingers held together, and perform a rhythmical clapping, alternately contacting the animal's chest and ribs. This is called "percussion" and sounds similar to a clip-clop of horse hooves. You may be wondering if I'm describing a type of hitting or striking on the chest, and yes, I am, but the cupping of the hands makes the contact comfortable for the patient. This curve of the hands also creates a mechanical force that helps to loosen lung fluids.

After a few minutes of percussion, the therapist performs a shaking technique to the ribcage, called "vibration," which further serves to move the loosened secretions into the larger airways, where the animal can cough and eliminate them from the lungs. The vibration is done by the therapist placing her hands flat, fingers together, on each side of the ribcage, then tightening her muscles and rapidly shaking the chest wall, similar to a trembling motion. The vibration technique is timed with the exhalation phase of breathing (as opposed to breathing in, or inhalation).

These techniques should only be done upon prior approval and medical clearance by the veterinarian.

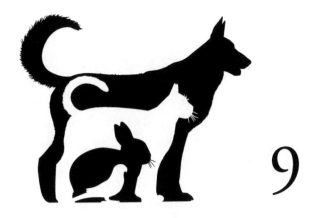

9

Performance Enhancement

Show Dogs

Dogs and other animals that participate in shows need to excel in their appearance, temperament, performance, obedience, and must conform to breed standards. They also need to be healthy and fit. Physical therapy plays a role in helping the dog achieve its maximum level of posture alignment, joint mobility, muscle length, strength, tone, and endurance. There must also be good communication between the therapist, owner, breeder, and handler, along with mutual respect. Physical therapists are knowledgeable and familiar with the basic standards of most breeds, but are not usually experts in the nuances of show terminology and technique. Although I have attended the Westminster Dog Show for many years, and most recently with media/press credentials that enabled me close access to all of the events, I still have a lot to learn. So, it is imperative that the owner, breeder, and handler provide the therapist with full disclosure of health history, their observations of abnormal movement, and any issues affecting a dog's performance in the ring. At that point, the therapist needs to be allowed to evaluate the dog, assess any problems, and formulate treatment intervention. I stress this as I have been on the receiving end of handlers, owners, and breeders "ordering" their dog's treatment, as if they are at the McDonald's drive-through window! Dog show competitions can be quite tense with so much at stake, but when cooperation and teamwork prevail, everyone wins.

Conformation dogs need to be outstanding examples of their breed and have good postural alignment, fluid movement, and high fitness levels. These are areas a physical therapist can help maximize through applications of modalities such as laser, electrical stimulation, massage, cold or hot packs, and techniques for stretching, joint mobilization, or manipulation. These are quick treatments that can be performed on-site at the benching areas at a show.

Therapists can also help troubleshoot any abnormal signs or issues that emerge in the ring and mitigate their potential development. Signs to be aware of that could signal strain, fatigue, or risk of an impending injury include a dog avoiding a particular activity or movement direction; yawning during event or practice sessions;

preferring to sit or lie down; running out of the rink and lacking normal level of obedience to its handler. Early recognition and intervention can be critical in the success of that day's showing. If the therapist is unable to be present at the event, you can make arrangements for communication via phone, Skype, picture, and video for assistance and recommendations.

Follow-up treatment can be combined with periods of rest for a week or two after a show in which a dog has signs of strain, sprain, or other injury. Your veterinarian should be consulted regarding any tests, medications, etc.

Physical therapists can also be utilized pre-show to help the dog prepare and maximize its fitness level two to three weeks before the event. Massaging, stretching, core training with a Physio-Roll, use of Cavaletti rails, swimming, leash walking, and trotting at various speeds and around obstacles help boost performance and prevent injury. When your dog feels its best during physical activity, its confidence and "sparkle" will be sure to catch the judge's discerning eye!

Agility

Agility activities and competitions are great forms of exercise and exciting for dogs and their human families. Certain canine breeds are naturally adept at mastering the negotiation of obstacles arranged in a course. Others need practice to develop and refine their skills. Agility courses require a high level of fitness, speed, and precision in turning, jumping, and landing. Jumping is an integral part of agility. Good jumping requires balance and accurate take-off. The take-off point and angle are very important as they determine the shape of the arc over the obstacle. Dog trainers, certified in agility, can be very helpful in teaching your dog the necessary strategy for these maneuvers through classes and clubs, using signals, voice, and movement commands.

Physical therapists, while not the best choice for training, can provide an integral service in the prevention of acute muscle strains or ligament sprains. Physical therapy can provide stretching to warm up and prepare these soft tissues to safely transition from a static still position to dynamic movement without injury. Muscle stretching in the agility athlete is also effective in achieving and maintaining an optimal muscle length to enhance performance. This occurs through the "length-tension relationship," in which the length of muscle fibers affects the force produced. There is an optimal point in a muscle's range of movement, at which it produces its maximal contractile tension. A muscle that is either too tight or overstretched will not produce an efficient contraction. A physical therapist has the knowledge and experience to help keep key muscle groups, needed for jumping, at their proper length.

Fitness level is the other area, essential to agility, that a physical therapist can help your dog optimize. It is best accomplished through cross-training and specificity. Cross-training uses a variety of aerobic exercises such as swimming, underwater or land treadmills, hiking, and jogging or trotting on level and uphill/downhill surfaces. Specificity refers to choosing activities that mimic movements performed during agility events. Balance exercises using wobble or rocker boards, core strengthening with Physio-Rolls, and toy and ball playing that incorporate turns, can all help achieve high levels of fitness. Currently no research exists to guide therapists and trainers on the correct amount of fitness training safe for dogs. However, the following is a general guide that can be modified depending on the dog's breed and natural athletic ability: up to one hour per day, up to six days per week of a combination of aerobic cross-training and functional /balance/core exercises. In addition to this, specific strengthening exercises using Thera Bands or weights for key muscle groups can be performed fifteen to twenty minutes, twice per week. Stretching can be provided two to three times per week for approximately ten to fifteen minutes. Regular leash walks should continue daily in addition to these activities. There should be one or two days per week that are resting, leash walk only days.

Puppies can participate in agility exercise and classes but my recommendation is to wait until they are older pups, at least nine months of age, when bone growth plates have closed. When in doubt, check with your veterinarian for best recommendations on growth plate maturation.

Keep in mind various body types and head shapes of dogs, when determining safe amounts of exercise and training. Chondrodystrophic or dwarf breeds, such as Dachshunds or Corgis, may need to avoid vertical jumps and sharp turns, but excel in speed walking and running exercises. Brachiocephalic or flat-faced breeds, such as Pugs or Boston Terriers, may do better with jumps and turns but need to avoid heavy durations of running due to their decreased cardiopulmonary capacity.

Sports

A great many sporting activities exist today for dogs and other species such as racing, flyball, hiking, carting, Frisbee, mushing, musical freestyle, and Treibball. As with human sports, animals get injured and require medical care along with physical therapy.

Injuries can occur with sporting activities from fractures, abrasions, tears, strains and sprains, dislocations, dehydration, skin lacerations, foot pad irritation, and nail trauma. Sesamoid disease is also common in sporting activity, involving the small round bones located in tendons and ligaments in the elbow, stifle, ankle (hock), and digits in the paws. The causes are usually due to intensity of performance, inadequate warm-up, trauma from direct contact, falling, or slipping.

Two types of sporting injury that are most challenging and require physical therapy are dislocations and instabilities. These are commonly seen in the canine shoulder and involve the joint capsule, ligaments, rotator cuff tendons, and cartilage. One injury in particular, medial shoulder instability, is performance-related, and thought to be secondary to excessive repetitive activity and overuse syndrome. This leads to persistent inflammation, degeneration of tissues, and lowering of tensile strength, which predisposes a joint to fray, breakdown, and leads to instability. The outward signs become apparent over time, and start to be noticed when the dog refuses to weave or turn a certain way or in a particular direction, with lameness on weight-bearing activity. Diagnosis is made by physical examination, radiograph, and MRI. In moderate to severe cases of instability, surgery, followed by physical therapy and rehabilitation, is the best treatment option. After surgery, a long rest period is required to allow the joint to start stabilizing. Interestingly, inflammation and scar tissue formation are desired as both are a crucial and a positive step in the healing process. This means that early physical therapy, normally desired after most orthopedic surgery in animals, is a bad idea here. Modalities such as laser and medications used for anti-inflammatory properties should not be used. Physical therapy should wait until six to eight weeks after the operation to allow tensile strength and protective scar tissue to develop, in order to stabilize the shoulder joint.

Custom shoulder supports (such as the Hobble, made by DogLeggs) are usually recommended three to four weeks post-op. Medication for pain (different from anti-inflammatory medication) will be prescribed, along with range of motion to the surrounding joints such as the elbow, carpus (wrist), digits, and the dog's neck. The shoulder should not be moved at this time, to allow for protective, good tightening to occur. You will be encouraged to begin taking your dog for slow leash walks, with the shoulder external supports in place.

At six to eight weeks post-operation, the therapist can start gentle range of motion to the shoulder joint, along with massage to decrease muscle spasm and functional electrical stimulation, to improve muscle bulk. Muscle strengthening exercises can begin at this time and rapid progression of full weight bearing on the forelimb, with the shoulder support used.

Over the eight to twelve weeks post-operation period, the external shoulder support can be used intermittently and weaned, according to the instructions given by the veterinary surgeon. Physical therapists should always defer to the advice of the surgeon regarding this critical item of weaning the support. The surgeon is the best person to make this decision.

Generally, the dog can return to full activity, including sports, in sixteen to twenty weeks post-operation. I'm sure it is pretty obvious that any effort to prevent this type of injury with its lengthy recovery and rehabilitation is highly valuable. Physical therapists can play an important role not only as rehabilitators, but also as providers of preventative interventions.

Examples of treatment interventions that can help to prevent repetitive injury are using modalities like laser and applications of cold packs to reduce swelling of tissues immediately after high intensity activity. Stretching before and after sports to target muscles, such as the psoas (hip flexor) and hamstrings, along with the Achilles tendon, can increase tissue length and reduce the potential for micro tears and strains. Core strengthening exercises can improve the dog's balance and control at the pivotal take-off points of jumps and turns, thus avoiding missteps or slips. Client education is also critical as the therapist can point out important signs to look for, spotting a potential problem early in the process before it leads to a serious injury. Cross-training is also important in reducing repetitive injury, so a therapist might recommend an alternate activity such as swimming. A simple suggestion by the therapist to rest the dog or reduce the frequency and intensity of sport activity for a temporary period might prevent a multitude of future days and hours of forced immobilization.

Another common sports injury in canines is strain of the hip flexor muscle, called "iliopsoas" or "psoas" for short. It is pulled, torn, or irritated during various highly active sporting events with jumps and turns, which tend to overextend it. Dogs with an injury to the psoas will display difficulty rising and have a short stride length during gait. It is diagnosed by palpation and use of thermal imaging. Technology for thermal imaging is available in some veterinary clinics to identify areas of inflammation and monitor its progression. It is treated with muscle relaxers and anti-inflammatory medications prescribed by your veterinarian, and physical therapy consisting of ice packs, laser, ultrasound, massage, gentle passive range of motion, Cavaletti rails, Physio-Rolls, and wobble boards. Stretching exercises should not be performed as they are contraindicated for this injury. Weave poles or figure-eight turns are also contraindicated.

(See Note 18.)

Earth and Working Activities

There is a certain joy that comes from watching a dog participate in activities that showcase its natural inherited ability. Examples of this are fielding, herding, hunting, tracking, retrieving, nose work, and Schutzhund (or for police work, search and rescue). These dogs tend to be courageous and focused on their purpose, performing their jobs with great enthusiasm. I have had the pleasure of working with Dash, a sheep-herding Border Collie; Lizzy, a herding Rottweiler; Raisin, a "go-to-ground" Border Terrier; Rex, a police K9 German Shepherd, and Penelope, my underground hunting and digging miniature Dachshund. Each of these dogs sustained injuries requiring PT: spine strains, hip muscle pulls from sprinting, cruciate ligament tears, cuts and lacerations, bites, paw pad injuries from navigating uneven terrain, and general trauma from an underground tunnel collapse. I do not mean to indicate that earth dog and working activity is dangerous, as I actually encounter more injuries with repetitive sports and agility courses. The nature of earth and working duties are vigorous and can be unpredictable with quite a mixed bag of injuries produced!

Physical therapy for these dogs is usually rehabilitative, post-injury or post-surgery. Raisin originally fell when she was a three-month-old puppy and sustained a fracture just below the stifle (knee), at the tibia, near her growth plate. Over time, a buttress of bony growth formed and eventually caused a shearing tear of her cranial cruciate ligament. She was very active in obedience and earth dog hunting competitions at the time, so her owner/parent Judy, was highly concerned about Raisin's future in these events. Raisin had lateral release CCL surgical repair with physical therapy starting two weeks after the operation. Raisin's natural obedience and cooperation, along with mom Judy's diligence in following the daily home exercise program, paid off royally. Raisin went back to competition and won veteran best of breed and first place in the veteran Terrier group, less than twenty weeks after her surgery!

Physical therapy can also play a role in injury prevention with endurance activities such as hiking, underwater treadmill walking and trotting, figure-eight turns around poles or cones focusing on tight, precise movements, walking up and down hills using voice commands or auditory signals for fast starts and stops, and holding a position midway down an incline. All of these activities and drills condition the dog not just in cardiovascular endurance, but also by stimulating the firing and timing mechanisms in the joint receptors. This helps their bodies adapt quickly to unexpected forces from uneven or shifting ground, etc.

Your veterinarian or physical therapist can also perform preventative exams every six months to check for joint integrity, tightness of muscles, posture and alignment, etc. Stretching, posture work, and mobilization of spinal or other joints can be provided in one to two sessions, to keep optimal physical condition for your active pet.

Walking as Therapy

What type of therapy do I mean? Physical? Emotional? Mental?

And the answer is: all of these! If you consider your dog to be a big part of your daily life, then time spent with it takes on great importance. One of the most valuable ways to enjoy your time together and accomplish great things for both of you is go on a leash walk!

Let's examine the benefits to you, the human person, first:

Dogs keep us focused on a daily routine and can be a powerful secret to productivity. On those days you dread getting started, you will always honor the commitment to get going and take care of your dog. After the morning outdoor business and feeding are completed, the walk begins. It stimulates both your and the dog's metabolic rate to ramp up. Simply participating in this normal rhythm of life will give you energy, meaning, and purpose to start your busy day. If you can return home during the day for a quick time-out to play and visit your dog, it provides a break from the grind. At the day's end, regardless of what has happened, your dog's greeting is always exuberant and helps you feel that life is still safe, just as you left it in the morning. It provides emotional well-being for both of you.

Dogs also play a role in improving our physical and mental health. Research shows that exercising with your dog can lower blood pressure. Studies involving patients with coronary artery disease show a pattern that those with pets were more likely to survive one year after an incident. This finding is strengthened by the fact that dog owners have the added benefit of more exercise through regular walks. Dog owners are considerably more likely to engage in moderate intensity walking three or more times per week, which results in a reduction of minor health problems.

Now, how about the benefits to your dog? Your dog loves time spent with you! The dog is a member of your family and has a natural instinct to be with its pack. Although the usual daily walks are one-on-one with you and your dog, I like to recommend that families take a group walk together with their dog at least once per week.

Start out with proper equipment such as a lead and harness or collar, pick-up bag, water, and pet ID. The dog should be tagged and micro-chipped. I also recommend having a photo of the dog carried in your pack, wallet, etc. Starting slow and gradually picking up the pace allows the muscles to warm up, the cardiopulmonary system to accommodate, and less stress on the paw pads. Go at a pace both of you can enjoy.

There are instances where you will need to do slower, controlled leash walks. These are important for more than canine good citizen manners. If your dog is starting leash walks after an injury or surgery, or has a chronic condition such as arthritis, it is important to do a slower, controlled speed of walking to allow maximum usage of the affected limb. A shorter lead should be used. If the dog is allowed to move too fast, it will spend less time on the limb during the stance phase of gait and hold the limb up longer during the swing phase. The dog will simply do what is easiest and hold the affected limb up, therefore not using it deliberately and compensating by overusing the sound limbs. Going slower will force the dog to touch down and push off from the affected limb, bearing more weight on that limb. Take breaks to allow your dog to reset its rhythm and avoid too much repetitive forces on its limbs and paws, especially if it is older or has chronic inflammatory conditions.

The result will be that your dog will gain more strength and build tissue bulk from previously atrophied musculature. This type of walk will be challenging and fun for both of you, serving as a positive reward during the recovery process.

If your dog is able to maintain good symmetry and equal use of the limbs during walking, you can add mini intervals of intensity, to increase its endurance and stimulate fat burning. These can be brief bursts of faster pace jogging or trotting, moving up and down small hills or inclines, or going up and down a few steps. I suggest these intervals to be between five and thirty seconds in duration, and be inserted three to four times during the course of your walk.

How long to walk? It is a difficult question to answer but in general, start with five to ten minutes if your dog has been injured or had surgery. Only progress the time if it is not limping and able to stay symmetrical, using both sides evenly at a controlled speed. You should be able to cover a quarter mile in about five minutes or a half mile in ten minutes for an average, moderate speed. When in doubt, you can always slow it down to a pace that covers a quarter mile in seven to eight minutes, for example. Work up gradually over the next few weeks to a good maintenance level of thirty to forty minutes of dog walking once per day, with a second shorter walk of ten to fifteen minutes.

For safety, pay attention to sounds and sights during the walk. Stay off cell phones, tablets, and avoid headphones. Keep a sharp eye out for dangers lurking in leaf piles or next to curbs that your dog might try to eat

BEST GUIDANCE
Your pet is capable of understanding much of what you say to it. If you need to correct its gait pattern, just say, "Okay, slow down," or "Easy now." If it needs to bear more weight on a limb, say, "Now put your foot down!" If it is knuckling and needs to put the paw flat, say, "Fix it!" If you say these commands with consistency in tone and rhythm, the pet will quickly pick up on what you wish it to do!

such as discarded food, candy, and bones. Avoid extremes in weather and watch for any signs of heatstroke: rapid breathing, drooling, stumbling, lethargy, bright redness of the gums and tongue, thick saliva, and vomiting. If this occurs, go to a shady area; apply cool water to the neck, face, and paws; assist or carry your dog to shelter; and contact the vet.

What does normal walking look like in a dog? Certain breeds have different patterns of locomotion. Generally, the walking gait is a four-beat pattern with three limbs on the ground at all times. The trot is a faster two-beat diagonal gait and the diagonal paws touch down at the same time. In other words, the right hind limb and the left front limb move together, and then the left hind limb moves with the right front. As the trot increases, it turns into a flying trot, and then a gallop. The flying trot is similar to the trot, but at a faster speed. The gallop, a four-beat gait is the fastest of all and is typically a quick right-left front limb, followed by nearly simultaneous but separate hind limb propulsion. Other mid-speed types of gait are the canter and pacing. The canter is a fast three-beat gait where two limbs move separately and the other two move as a diagonal pair. Pacing is a two-beat gait where one side of the body's limbs move in pair, followed by the other side. The left front and rear limbs move at the same time, followed by the right front and rear limbs.

(See Note 19.)

Injury Prevention

Physical therapy plays a huge role in prevention, wellness, weight management, and fitness. Early use of PT after an injury or surgical procedure can reduce abnormal scar tissue formation, promote proper postural alignment, and prevent future arthritic conditions or wear/tear on joints and tendons. A good therapist can also teach valuable ways to prevent problems as your dog ages; for example, starting core strengthening exercises and training in use of a ramp for a young Dachshund to avoid future spinal issues.

Loving pet owners everywhere share a common concern in keeping their animals healthy, happy, and safe. We go to great lengths to provide proper nutrition, medical care, fun activity, and shelter. When problems occur, we provide the necessary resources to insure our pets' needs are met. Wouldn't it feel great to also provide safeguards to actually prevent injury from occurring? Imagine the ability to have more control in helping your pet stay healthier, reducing financial costs of treatment and care, and overall peace of mind. All it takes is a bit of knowledge, a few modifications, and some helpful insight from a friend (me!) who has been on the frontlines treating injured pets.

Here are my best suggestions for injury prevention:

1. Know thy breed: If you have a pure breed pet you need to research the details of the normal traits and conformation as well as medical conditions specific to that breed. For example, Dachshunds and other short-limb canines are susceptible to spinal injuries. Great Danes and Weimaraners tend to develop neck instabilities such as Wobbler syndrome. Cats and canine toy breeds often have difficulty with luxating patella. Shepherds, Saint Bernards, and Rottweilers, tend to develop hip dysplasia. Good sources of information include your veterinarian, breeder, blogs such as *Dawg Business: It's Your Dog's Health*, books, and the Internet. If your pet

is a mixed breed, you can still be guided by the general characteristics of the primary breeds that are apparent visually or by DNA testing. You can also take some measure of comfort that mixed breeds offer in terms of genetic diversity, being less likely to express some of the above disorders or in lesser degrees than a pure bred pet.

2. Maintain a reasonable weight: Your pet does not have to be thin, just within a fairly normal range for its breed and size. Let your veterinarian guide you accordingly. Along with body weight, keeping good muscle tone is important. A physical therapist can show you some simple exercises and activities to maximize strength. Keeping excess body weight off the joints, ligaments, and tendons will help avoid arthritis, sprains and strains, and aggravation of hip or elbow dysplasia. Good muscle strength and tone also de-loads and supports joints.

3. Hardwood, tile, or other slippery floors and surfaces are the enemy! I cannot stress enough how dangerous slippery surfaces are for causing cruciate ligament tears and soft tissue strains. Many families love the look of hardwood floors and have it throughout their homes. They also feel wood floors are cleaner and don't absorb stains and odor. These positives are outweighed by the negatives in terms of potential canine injury. The solution is to use area rugs over the hardwood in large rooms and carpet runners in hallways and on stairs. Avoid small throw rugs, as they can be slippery as well. Garage and outdoor deck wood steps should be equipped with

nonskid pads. In terms of the outdoors, be mindful to keep your dog off slippery wet grass unless it is on leash. Avoid having your dog run or walk on ice or slush. Snow and sand are usually safe for dogs to walk, run, and play in, but use common sense on the duration of activity.

4. Minimize the jumping on/off furniture: Do whatever you can to minimize or restrict this, such as blocking furniture with large pillows, depending on your particular pet. Larger pets can easily climb on and off of furniture without danger of injury. The act of jumping, particularly down rather than up, causes shearing force on the knee ligaments, and jarring to the forelimb elbow and wrist joints, and the spine. In my experience, most pets don't use those little steps you can buy to climb up and down from the bed. The best solution is a ramp, preferably lined with carpet or a non-stick pad and built-up sides. Use a leash to train your pet to use the ramp. If the pet senses the ramp is sturdy, it should have no problem using it. Sometimes a little ingenuity is needed and if you are handy, consider building one yourself. My engineer husband built one for our Dachshund, complete with a hinge to fold it up and store under the couch when company comes! Use gates or other ways to block staircases.

5. Keep up grooming: Keep your pet's nails trimmed, pads moisturized, and hair between the paw toes clipped, to allow proper weight bearing and distribution during walking, play, and standing. This is one of the easiest and most effective ways of avoiding injury.

6. Take it easy: Avoid heavy play with other pets, or with the pet's parents! Ball play doesn't need to be a high intensity activity. If your pet loves to lunge and play hard, just moderate the duration and frequency of such activity.

7. Variety is the spice of life: Exuberance can cause excessive running around in circles, sudden twists and turns that can cause acute strains. The best way to avoid this is by keeping your pet stimulated and not bored, by rotating toys, varying activity or environment, and taking it for regular controlled leash walks. Simply letting the pet out in the yard does not provide variety or stimulation. Leash walking in the neighborhood or in parks and on trails allows it to sniff and explore, receive message signals, and provides mental and physical stimulation. Exuberance is wonderful but it is much safer to spread out the happiness through a variety of activity, to lessen those over-the-top spurts.

8. Encourage spay/neuter: Readers of this book are already fully aware of the reasons for spay and neutering, from prevention of certain diseases to the dangers of close breeding practices resulting in unnecessary deformities. I am currently working with an adorable dog, obtained from a retail pet store, who had already endured three orthopedic surgeries before the age of eighteen months. He is the product of careless, for-profit breeding, and is at risk for future arthritis and pain, hopefully minimized by having PT.

Core Strengthening

In the event you might research canine or pet strengthening, part of the new field of PT and rehabilitation for animals, you will find plenty of information about the fore and hind limbs. You will not find much at all on the core groups that contain the diaphragm, abdominal, and spinal musculature. As time goes on, we realize just how critical these muscle groups are to animal function and the importance of properly including them in a rehabilitation program. The abdominal muscles are those that run from the ribs to parts of the pelvis. Their names are rectus abdominus, external and internal obliques, and transverse abdominus. Their functions are 1) movement (bending or flexion, side bend, and rotation of the spine); 2) support for the spine and visceral organs; and 3) to assist or act as an accessory to activity, breathing, and barking. The rectus is superficial and runs long ways in a head-to-tail direction (like the six-pack stomach muscle in the human); the obliques are diagonal, along the pet's side; and the transverse is a deep, lower muscle that runs from side to side. When you visualize how the pet walks in a quadruped (all four limbs on the ground) manner with its internal organs positioned parallel to the ground, you can see how important the abdominal muscles are in providing a type of floor support to counter the effects of gravity. Canines also have a much shorter gut/intestinal path as compared to humans, and the abdominals can be helpful in aiding this system.

It is important to strengthen and firm the abdominals muscles for prevention of spinal conditions in dogs, particularly the chondrodystrophic (dwarf) breeds like Dachshunds, Corgis, Pekingese, and Lhasa Apsos, or after spinal injury or spinal surgery. In non-orthopedic cases where abdominal surgery is performed for removal of masses, etc., the abdominal area will need rehabilitation to help tissue healing and regain strength.

Typical PT intervention after abdominal surgery will include massage over the surgery site. Abdominal incisions are deep and tend to form excess scar tissue. This forms naturally as the body heals itself and it usually reabsorbs with normal movement and activity. However, sometimes excess scarring can linger and impair muscle function. These cross links of excess collagen are broken down through various types of massage. The most common is transverse friction, where a shearing type of movement is performed perpendicular to the scar direction (e.g., if scar runs north-south, the friction is applied east-west). Another form is myofascial release, a very light, subtle rhythmical surface technique that works on the fascia or connective tissues surrounding the musculature. There are other somatic body work vibratory techniques used by massage therapists that can also help. In the human PT world, the Wurn Technique is used over the abdominal region to release scar tissue in women having difficulty conceiving. I anticipate these techniques may eventually become adapted for use in animals having medical abdominal issues.

Now for the fun part! Here are some examples of strengthening and toning exercises:

1. Get on the ball: Using a peanut-shaped ball or Physio-Roll, place the pet on top, long ways, and perform gentle bouncing motions, while keeping one hand on your dog and one on the ball. This will activate and recruit the abdominal musculature.

2. Sit up for a treat: This exercise can be performed starting with your dog lying on its back. A pillow or mattress can be placed underneath. Place one hand under its ribs or behind the neck, while the other hand holds a small treat, and then encourage the dog to do a curl- or sit-up and reach for the treat. This engages the rectus muscle, by working from the top down. Five reps.

3. Add a twist: Roll your dog toward its side using a cushion or pillow under the ribs and do the same sit-up as above, but from the side, to activate the obliques. Repeat on the other side. Three to four reps per side.

4. Bottoms up: Now work from the bottom up to recruit the deeper transverse abdominals. Start with the dog on its back. Lean over the dog and tickle its lower belly, rub your head on the fur, or something similar that is fun for your dog, so it will naturally want to curl-up its legs and bottom. This is not done in reps but in time. Try to make this a fun little game, getting the dog to hold the position for ten to fifteen seconds. My dog likes when my hair falls down on her belly!

5. Belly tickle: If your dog has difficulty lying on his back or side for the above exercises, you can start with a basic belly tickle in the standing-on-all-fours position. Place one hand under its chin to align the head horizontally, and the other hand lightly tickling the belly to encourage abdominal muscular contraction.

6. Stretching: Like all muscles, the abdominals can get tight and may need to be stretched. This should be done by a PT or your vet, via rolling from side to side and lying back over a small rolled towel or foam roller.

General precautions and contraindication: Though I love to provide examples of PT exercises for you to do at home, the safest and best way is to be shown first by an animal-trained PT or a rehab-trained vet. They can provide specific modifications and parameters for the best outcome. I would avoid abdominal strengthening in certain high-cut/deep-chested breeds such as boxers as there may be a risk of stimulating gastric torsion. It is always best to get your vet's advice first. Have a great time and help firm your pet's abs!

(See Note 20.)

The Tables Are Turned

After all of this talk on performance enhancement for our pets, allow me to turn the tables a bit and focus on how pets enhance our human performance. You already know about animals used in service, helping the blind and deaf, being therapy pets in nursing homes and developmental centers, but did you know that animals are now being used as assistants in human physical therapy and rehabilitation?

Yes, animals partner with physical and occupational therapists in helping human patients to relearn task sequencing by brushing their coats, applying collars and harnesses, feeding them, etc. Strengthening is accomplished by having a human patient reach up or out to touch and pet an animal, or place it on the lap or up on a perch, etc. Physical therapists use dogs to assist with gait training for patients after a stroke or with Parkinson's to provide help with balance as well as promoting mobility. Dogs have an innate sense of when to slow down and accommodate to a person's special needs, similar to how a dog knows to be gentle around a baby or toddler. Speech language pathologists use animals to help patients vocalize and verbalize. Children receive help in developing their speaking skills by reading aloud to attentive animals.

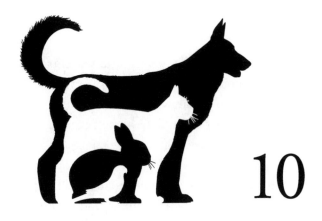

10

Expectations of Care

Maintenance

"No pain, no gain" is a common slogan used to depict rehabilitation and physical therapy. Yet physical therapy does not
have to be painful and is not always used for gain. There are
many roles a physical therapist plays in the health care field,
among which is in maintenance of function and well-being.
Ironically, in human medicine the concept of maintenance is
poorly received and barely reimbursed by third-party insurance
carriers. Most, if not all, insurance carriers will pay only on
claims that show patient improvement and deny claims that
show a lack of progress. There should be more value placed on
treatment interventions that offer alternative outcomes, such as
disease prevention and prevention of disease progression. Thus,
maintenance care in physical therapy serves to reduce the possibility of future decline in patients, both human and animal! For
animals, maintenance physical therapy is valuable in conditions
such as chronic degenerative arthritis, neuromuscular disease,

partial cruciate ligament tears, intervertebral disc bulge's, congenital joint laxity, etc. Upon completion of a successful physical therapy program where the long- and short-term goals have been reached, or met to the highest expected degree, many pet owners choose to continue the treatment on a maintenance basis, to ensure their pets stay safe and are able to function at the same level. Although a home program will be provided and continued by the pet owner, some aspects of care such as joint mobilization, laser, and massage techniques cannot be easily duplicated and the services of a professional can fill that gap. I recommend a frequency of one maintenance visit every three to four weeks for periodic monitoring and treatment, with the goal of stabilizing the animal's status. If this seems to be working well after a few sessions, the interval can be increased to one maintenance visit every four to six weeks. I have not had good results using an interval wider than six weeks, without risking going back to square one with therapy intensity. The mainte-nance therapy model is also beneficial to pets that need more intervention than chemical only or those that cannot tolerate long-term use of medications due to side effects. Maintenance is also budget friendly and a cost savings when compared to allowing a condition to worsen, requiring expensive tests and follow-up later on.

Supportive

When a medical condition is progressive and results in a steady decline, treatment interventions are termed as "supportive." Physical therapy can play a role in these cases, by providing tem-porary relief of pain, reducing complications and side effects, giving comfort, and maximizing the pet's quality of daily life.

Such conditions that might require supportive therapy are: cancers, Cushing's, advanced degenerative myelopathy, and other metabolic or medical diseases that cannot be cured. Physical therapy should not utilize any modality that could exacerbate or worsen a condition, such as use of ultrasound or laser over a cancerous tumor, and all pertinent medical history should be disclosed before treatment begins. Gentle massage, range of motion, Reiki, light exercises, and functional activities can be part of a supportive physical therapy treatment, provided in a clinic or in-home setting. The frequency of care is variable, depending on the animal's response, particular medical needs, and economic considerations.

It is also important to note that the effects of physical therapy are not just physical, but can enhance a pet's emotional and social well-being also. It can help a pet suffering from cognitive or mental issues, by supporting the medical care of such conditions. This is similar to human psychiatric conditions that are often managed by use of medication plus talk therapy or psychotherapy. Veterinary behaviorists, along with animal trainers, animal communicator, and possibly pet psychics are helpful in providing the emotional and therapeutic elements of psychotherapy. Physical therapy can be of further use, providing results that are similar to the relaxation a human gets from having a massage or the stress release from walking and exercising. I became familiar with this concept during my volunteer work in an animal shelter with dogs that had endured abuse and neglect. Our zoo director and chief veterinarian would often ask me to work with these dogs to help instill a sense of security and comfort. Though there were no objective physical deficits to address, I was able to apply simple handling, positioning, range of motion, massage, leash walking and trotting, and simple human-animal contact, with soothing words and songs, etc. This seemed to unlock anxiety and help the dogs regain their confidence and trust. The results were consistently positive in two or three sessions, showing increased interactions, making eye contact, and relaxation of facial grimacing or tension.

Standards of Practice

Currently there are no documented consistent standards of practice for providers of animal physical therapy and rehabilitation. However, if your provider is a licensed physical therapist and belongs to the American Physical Therapy Association (APTA), she must adhere to a Code of Ethics and Guide to Professional Conduct in order to maintain membership. There are also licensure regulations that physical therapists and veterinarians must adhere to but they are not nationalized and vary from state to state.

Here is a sample list of the type of standards found in the APTA documents mentioned above, that therapists should follow:

- Core values of accountability, altruism, compassion, excellence, integrity, professional duty, and even social responsibility.
- Ethical behavior and how it can be challenged in various practice environments where PT services are provided.
- Respect for the rights, privacy, and dignity of all patients.
- Exercise sound judgments that are within the therapist's scope of practice and level of expertise and in the patient's best interest.

- Continuous learning and lifelong acquisition of knowledge and skills.
- Promoting and ensuring safety in all work environments.
- Trustworthiness and protection of the public from incompetent or illegal acts.

In order to feel comfortable that your provider is committed to a high standard of practice, you might ask to see her license or certification, along with asking what professional associations she belongs to. In some states, it is required by law that licensure or certification documents be posted in an area the consumer can easily see. If care is being provided in your home, the therapist should carry a wallet-sized document of her license.

An ethical provider will always make decisions based on the medical need of your pet and not on monetary gain. She will be committed to the least amount of care needed to attain the highest results. In other words, she should never overtreat the patient.

Frequency of care should be determined according to what will best benefit the animal. During the initial or acute phase of care, visits may be twice per week and very occasionally three times per week. Animals tend to respond quickly to physical therapy and hold the improvement for a longer period of time compared to human beings, so this intensity of care is usually very short. After many years of providing PT to the human population, I have been able to compare the response to PT in animals and have found it to be consistently faster. Animals are very accepting of their circumstances and have fewer barriers to cross. They love human contact and readily absorb the therapeutic benefits of PT. Within about two weeks, treatment can be reduced to a frequency of one or two times per week. When the animal demonstrates significant improvement and the owner can handle some of the exercises at home, frequency is further reduced to every other week.

The length of each treatment session: The initial visit will last sixty to ninety minutes, including the evaluation, home program instruction, and some treatment. The follow-up treatment sessions can run between thirty to sixty minutes, depending on the type of animal. For example, a feline case may be shorter in length due to the smaller body size and nature of injury a cat usually presents with. On average, a visit will last forty-five to fifty minutes.

Fees

Currently, the general range of fees for an initial evaluation session runs between $75 and $150. I am aware of some facilities that charge as high as $200. For a follow-up treatment session you can expect to pay between $50 and $110, with some facilities charging as much as $125.

Fees will range depending on the geographic region and type of facility or particular level of expertise offered. Ultimately, you as a consumer will be the one to decide if the fees charged are reasonable and deserved compared to the care being given.

Most veterinarians and physical therapists are not heavily schooled in business management, but they consult with an accountant or other professional to determine an appropriate fee schedule. Fees should be based on a careful calculation of the cost of providing care, plus a fair profit margin of 25 to 35 percent, for example. A fee should not be based on licking a finger and holding it up to find the wind, calling around to find out what other offices charge, or seeing how much people are willing to pay for their pet's care.

Many providers will expect fee for service, or payment in full at the time of the visit. Most offices will accept credit and debit card payments, in addition to cash and checks. Be sure to ask how your personal information, such as bank account and credit/debit card number, is protected against identity theft. The HIPPA (Health Insurance Privacy and Portability Act) privacy and protection laws originating from Department of Health and Human Services do not apply to veterinary practices at this time. However, most reputable veterinary physical therapy practices strive to model their office procedures accordingly.

Pet insurance usually covers a portion of physical therapy and rehabilitative care with a dollar limit per visit or per case. Check your specific policy to learn about specific coverage limits. The therapist might accept assignment, and submit a bill for service directly to your insurance carrier, waiting to be paid by the insurance company when the claim is processed. Most, however, will expect payment from you first, and provide a receipt or billing statement that you can submit to your insurance carrier for reimbursement. If the claim form has a section asking for clinical data, it is reasonable for you to ask the therapist to fill it in or help you complete this, without any additional charge.

Discount programs may be available in some facilities, where a nominal fee is charged per year, in exchange for a percentage (usually 15 to 25 percent) discount applied to any care needed. Payment plans might also be available through the facility or outside credit programs such as Care Credit.

Financial hardship should always be considered in planning care. If your pet needs physical therapy and you have

BEST GUIDANCE
"There are a great many things now taking place in veterinary medicine. I strongly suggest that all pet owners stay abreast of new trends in medicine. Sometimes medical practitioners are like wheelbarrows—they're useful tools, but they need to be pushed. Very often, educated owners can bring out the best in a vet." —Warren Eckstein

difficulty paying for it, be up front with your provider. Although they are under no obligation to reduce a fee, most will be willing to consider your particular circumstances. You may be asked to show proof of income in some form if a sliding scale of fees exists for cases of documented financial hardship. If fees are not flexible or negotiable, ask if care can be provided less frequently and a home program be given.

Pro bono (free) or heavily discounted care should be provided to animal patients residing in shelters, humane societies, and rescue facilities or foster homes whenever possible.

Communication Between You, the Therapist, and Veterinarian

How to communicate? Let me count the ways…face-to-face, email, phone, fax, Skype, mail, and on and on. There is no bad form of communication, only bad if there is a lack of it!

Let's start with you and your pet's therapist: you should have a comfortable rapport and complete ease interacting together. A therapist must have great analytical problem-solving ability and excellent treatment skills but ultimately have the ability to work well with animals.

Your pet should sense the therapist's passion for it and respond to her voice and touch, but it may not be immediate. An animal may be a bit unsure the first few minutes, but will soon figure it out and understand that the therapist is there to help it. Animals cannot be fooled and they always recognize trained hands and genuine intent. If it is a good fit, they will trust the PT and enjoy the treatment sessions. Your pet's therapist should also have good interaction with the whole family: not just the humans but all of the animal members too! If other household pets that are normally shy come around to check things out and stay nearby, not simply for protection but by assuming a relaxed position, it is a sign that you have selected a wonderful therapist. One of the best experiences for a therapist is being surrounded by the other dogs, cats, and other family while rendering care to her patient.

As the pet's owner, please get involved: try to be present during the sessions, help with positioning, and stay close to be able to touch and pet them. Be aware that physical therapists are not trainers or animal control specialists, so don't expect expert advice on behavior or discipline, and be prepared to assist with making sure your pet is able to cooperate and tolerate the care for optimum results.

Feel free to ask questions, and communicate between therapy sessions if the need arises. You may have to wait for a return phone call or email, but it should be handled within twenty-four hours or less. Physical therapists tend to be friendly folks and good listeners, but also quite busy, so try to keep your conversations succinct.

A medical record, hard copy or electronic, will be established for your pet with each therapy session, documented in terms of medical history, initial evaluation, follow-up session dates, treatments provided, changes in status, outcomes, etc. The physical therapist should have a written program for your pet within seventy-two hours of the initial visit, which includes long- and short-term goals that are specific and measureable, a prognosis for completing the goals, and a description of the treatment plan. This report should be sent to your veterinarian and a copy to you. The report should be discussed with you and any questions answered, especially explanations of medical terminology. Follow-up communication on your pet's progress should be done at approximately three-week intervals, by phone, email, or fax, and copied to you.

Communication between the therapist and veterinarian should be bathed in mutual respect. There should be no competition between the two individuals. The veterinarian is the authority in medical care of animals and the physical therapist is an expert in physical rehabilitation. Each should rely on the other's experience and judgment and ultimately collaborate for the benefit of you and your precious animal.

Home Programs

Home programs include any special instructions, activities, treatments, or exercises that can be followed at home on a daily basis, between therapy sessions. The program should be demonstrated and given to you in writing, along with contact information if questions should arise before the next appointment. The therapist should give you some home exercises and instructions on the first visit and ensure that you have full understanding and capability to carry them out. In my experience, many pet owners are uncomfortable with handling an incision or moving a limb involving joint movements out of fear they will hurt the pet. If you are not at ease with any request in the home program, you must be candid with the therapist. She will appreciate your honesty and be able to make changes or substitutions to achieve the same or similar benefit. Adequate time and patience should be used in establishing a home program, as it is essential to good care. Pet owners who are compliant with follow-through of home programs are likely to enjoy greater and faster results of therapy.

If a particular item in the program is more complex, ask the therapist if you can take notes on the sheet, writing descriptions in your own handwriting or style of language that will help you remember the details later. Cell devices that capture video can also be taken to have a visual guide as well. If video is taken, do not post it online without obtaining permission from the therapist.

Outcomes and Discharge

You should expect the best possible care with maximum results, in the quickest time frame. The results should extend beyond basic recovery and into a renewed exuberance for life. When your pet begins to feel better physically, it is more likely to interact with the family, bring its toys out to play, and resume its former jobs such as protecting you or patrolling the yard and property borders.

Every therapist has her own work style and personality, but all should put forth diligent effort to ensure that the PT goals are met and within a reasonable amount of time. You should feel a connection with the clinician and observe a bond she shares with your pet. Most therapists are too busy to waste your time and will work productively to ensure good progress.

Their reputation is based on professionalism, ethics, and results! However, as the field of physical therapy and rehabilitation for animals grows and becomes more accessible to the consumer, the temptation for some to milk it may occur. You will sense if this is happening. So will your pet! Animals not only recognize skilled, trained hands, but also your intent and purpose. You already know they are great judges of character!

Allow me to insert a little story about a canine patient I was trying to discharge from therapy.

Cooper is a four-year-old white-coated Golden Retriever who had cruciate ligament tears in both of his knees and required surgery on each, only three weeks apart. This was quite disabling and caused him great difficulty with walking, climbing stairs, and standing. He began a program of canine swimming that helped him a lot, but his walking was still labored, with the hind limbs bent and crossed underneath him. Physical therapy was recommended and Cooper's mom Kathy got in touch with me to arrange treatment. She further enticed me by sending a short video of her adorable canine boy, struggling along the sidewalk awkwardly. He stole my heart and I was motivated to offer as much help to him as I could.

The rehabilitation process lasted seven months, with one-hour sessions each visit. I worked with Cooper in his home, surrounded by his loving family of three generations. Each week, Cooper gave it his all and the family cheered him on! We kept a chart of his progress with range of motion, measured in degrees, plus bulk of the leg muscles using a tape measure, his standing height, etc. We watched him steadily improve and reach the pre-set goals. Gradually I was able to reduce the frequency of PT from weekly to every other week, then every three weeks, and finally a month. On the last visit when I returned after a month, I found that not only had Cooper maintained all of his gains, but that he had further improved in standing taller with straighter hind legs, and with his ability to walk.

When the session ended I went into the kitchen to talk with his mom Kathy and give her my ecstatic news that Cooper was ready to be discharged. All of her time, effort, money, had paid off! As we were discussing this, Kathy's sister Linda quietly tiptoed over, tapped each of us on the shoulder simultaneously, and pointed to the dog, silently mouthing the words: *"Look at Cooper."* We turned to find Cooper sitting in the doorway of the kitchen with his head slumped completely down, resting on his chest. At first, I thought he must be sleeping, sitting up! I went over, bent down to look and his eyes were open, but very sullen. He looked completely despondent. His head stayed drooped but his eyes looked at me as if to say "Are you kidding me?" I went back to Kathy but before I could say a word, she quickly muttered, "Can you come back in six weeks?" "What day, what time?" came my reply. As we scheduled another session for Cooper, we heard him walk away, followed by a familiar thumping sound. She looked around the corner into the living room and there was Cooper in his bed, lying on his side with his tail wagging, with each beat hitting the floor. Kathy said to me, "Well, he knows you'll be coming back, and since he has another appointment, he is happy!"

I smiled, shook my head in amazement, went over, bent down, and gave the dog a pat on his head saying, "Okay, Coop. See you in a few weeks. Be a good boy!"

If you are being asked to schedule a greater-than-needed number or frequency of visits, be wary. Therapists should never base recommendations on producing revenue, making lease payments on expensive equipment, or paying rent on their building.

Discharge, or ending treatment, should be based on your pet's achieving the goals set or receiving the maximum benefit from therapy. The clinician will re-evaluate your pet's progress every few visits and review the goals to see if they are being met. If there is no change after two to three visits, the treatment should be modified to obtain a better response. Performing the same treatment over and over, without finding improvement in the animal, should prompt you to question the value of therapy.

In some instances, the goals will not be fully met due to unanticipated events or other factors that could not be predicted. In these cases, the therapist will need to determine why the goals could not be met and that all possible treatment approaches were utilized. If it is found that the maximum possible improvement has been achieved, then treatment will be discontinued. An exception to this would be if professional care is needed to maintain the goals, beyond what the family or owners are capable of providing on their own.

A therapist can discharge your pet from treatment if she feels the animal poses a danger or threat. This is a sensitive area and should be handled appropriately. Every effort must be made to ease tensions and adapt techniques so that intervention will be successful. There are some instances when, regardless of the therapist's attempt to modify a treatment approach, the animal does not tolerate therapy and treatment must be stopped. The need to discontinue is usually obvious to both the therapist and pet owner. An open discussion should occur along with suggestions made by the therapist for some sort of continuing care given by the owner or another qualified professional. Both parties should remain respectful of each other and ultimately hold the animal's concerns in the highest regard.

You as the pet owner can discharge treatment at any time and for any reason. You may not like the therapist after a session or two or be unhappy with results, etc. In this instance, the best way to sever the relationship is by simple but polite, honest communication.

Finally, there is the issue of patient abandonment, or an unexpected loss of service to your pet. This can occur from a multitude of reasons but most likely a medical emergency, temporary disability, a maternity or paternity leave, etc. Whenever possible, adequate warning or notice should be given. If that is not possible, then barring the death or mental incapacity of the therapist, alternate recommendations must be made so that the pet has continuity of care. As professionals, therapists keep a resource listing of local and regional care providers they can refer to in these types of situations. If you encounter any situation where you feel abandoned by a therapist and have no direction of where to seek alternative care, contact your veterinarian, state veterinary or physical therapy credentialing board, or local vet/PT association for assistance. In addition, you can ask to speak to a consumer advocate if you feel the need to document a complaint.

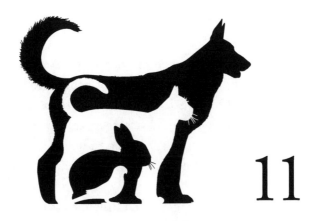

11

Other Related Topics

Splints, Wraps, and Braces

Let's start with braces, called "orthotics" in the medical world. A brace is made by a professional orthotist. Your veterinarian or therapist may recommend the use of a brace for your pet, based on a number of factors. Braces are generally used for three purposes:

1. Prophylaxis: for protection; used in conditions such as a dropped or paralyzed paw or limb that drags, knuckles over, and needs support to prevent abrasions, infection, etc.

2. Rehabilitative: to support a limb or body part while the animal is recovering from surgery or injury, such as a stifle brace after cranial cruciate ligament repair or a spinal brace to stabilize a fracture of the spine. In cases of torn cruciate ligaments, braces can be used after surgery

as an adjunct, if the animal needs additional support due to having a large body frame or being involved in very active sports. Cruciate rehabilitation braces are also used for pets that cannot have surgery due to advanced age, inability to tolerate anesthesia, or financial issues. These orthoses allow the stifle joint to flex and extend through the needed range of motion while helping to prevent the tibia from shifting or translating forward on the femur, acting as the ligament would if it were still intact.

3. Functional: to assist during functioning by providing support for long-term, chronic conditions. Examples of this might be to control range of motion in a joint that is floppy or unstable from a birth defect, also called "congenital anomaly," commonly seen in the carpal (wrist) joints; a torn Achilles tendon that results in a dropped hock; a joint or body part that has degenerative arthritis with painful erosion of cartilage and needs external support to de-load and relieve discomfort.

The fabrication of a brace starts with a cast of your pet's body part, which is usually done by a veterinarian or therapist with casting experience, and sent to the orthotist. The orthotist makes a positive mold or impression from the cast, to simulate the pet's limb. Specialized plastic material is formed over the mold, and then it is lined with foam products. Lightweight metal upright bars are placed on the inner and outer surfaces of the brace, with hinges at the joints. The hinges can be left open to allow full movement or locked to restrict it. There are also adjustable hinges to allow variable, controlled range of motion. Finally, the orthotist will configure any type of suspension needed to control the position of the brace on the limb, by use of straps, slings, Velcro, or other closures. If the pet has a shortened limb, a lift can be added to the paw plate to create extra length. When the brace is finished, it will be delivered or shipped to you, your veterinarian, or therapist. Before the pet starts wearing the brace, fit and alignment need to be checked out by the therapist. You will then be advised how to apply the brace and instructed on the number of hours on and off for wearing time. The first few days are critical for frequent removal and checking for skin abrasion or any abnormal signs of wear or irritation. A custom-fabricated brace can be sent back to the orthotist for adjustments and modifications as needed.

There are prefabricated braces also available that are less expensive than custom-made orthoses. Casting is not necessary for theses braces, and simple measurements can be taken by the pet owner or therapist to determine size. Prefabricated braces are available off the shelf and by order, but they do not always offer a perfect fit and cannot be modified.

Splints

Splints are lighter in weight and material in comparison to braces. They are used for support, stabilization, and stretching purposes. Splints are less expensive than braces and can be fabricated by a physical or occupational therapist or veterinarian. The therapist will make a blueprint on paper, drawing around your pet's limb or body part that requires the splint, outlining the shape and size. She will cut the drawing (similar to cutting out paper dolls) and trace it onto a sheet of low temperature thermoplastic material, leaving an additional one- to two-inch border. This material will be heated by immersing it in hot water to soften it, then taken out and cut to the proper shape, while it is malleable. A protective stocking should be placed on the pet's limb, and then the heated plastic is draped and molded on the animal. The plastic will cool and set within a few minutes. From that point, it is trimmed and fine-tuned using a heat gun or hot water to finish the edges and make any final adjustments. Padded lining will be added along with Velcro closures and straps. Extra padding or special cut-outs may be needed for bony areas or fragile, delicate skin conditions.

Splints can be a great help for support and protection of weakened joints such as the carpus and hock, or after muscle and tendon repairs. Splints can be converted from being simple static ones to dynamic by building small extensions called "outriggers," which hold elastic bands that can be looped around a floppy paw or toes, to prevent dragging. Other uses for dynamic splints are to correct muscle and joint contractures by providing a low-load tension that gives a prolonged stretch to joints such as the stifle, elbow, and carpus.

One drawback of splints is that they can be chewed by your pet. Vet wrap may need to be applied around the splint initially or a head cone used, along with monitoring.

Wraps

Wraps offer great solutions for support and shock absorption of joints and weakened areas, especially with lighter, smaller-framed animals. Larger animals can also benefit from wraps if only mild support is needed or for use during light activities. Wraps can also be used during sports, to add extra protection to a specific body part and provide heat and support.

Sometimes it can be difficult to determine whether a brace, splint, or wrap is needed, but your therapist or veterinarian can evaluate and make the best recommendations. Wraps are typically manufactured and sold by commercial pet industry retailers, especially the prefabricated type. Custom wraps are available from specialized vendors such as orthotists and occupational therapists. Wraps do not require cast molds or traced drawings, but simple measurements taken with a ruler or tape measurer. Measurements for prefabricated wraps can easily be taken by the pet owner. Custom wraps are best measured by a trained therapist, due to the precision needed in identifying anatomical landmarks, etc. Wraps are made from specialized fabric and neoprene, in light, moderate, and heavy weights relating to the type of joint support needed. Nylon support straps and padding can be added to give additional support or to limit movement and for protection.

I have ordered and used custom wraps for many of my animal patients, including dogs, cats, and goats, with great success. Examples are:

1. Kermit, a Pit Bull puppy with congenital joint laxity and hyperextended carpus joints, causing him to stand flat on the full paw. Custom carpal wraps were ordered and used during play and leash walking to support the wrist joints while he grew and matured skeletally and during his strengthening exercises in therapy. Wraps were a good choice as they offered flexibility and room to grow, as Kermit was only six months old. After six weeks, Kermit became stronger and was able to be weaned from the wraps, but they offered great protection of his joints during the transition process.

2. Sam, a two-year-old Pit Bull, was hit by a car and had sciatic nerve damage with dropped paw on the rear limb. The veterinarian determined that the nerve damage was likely temporary, so a tarsal/ankle wrap was chosen that extended up toward the knee and had elastic tension straps to hold the paw up and prevent dragging. Physical therapy consisted of functional electrical stimulation, ROM, and strengthening exercises, plus leash walking with the wrap support. Sam eventually had 80 percent of full nerve recovery and did not need the wrap for activity in the home, but continued to use it during longer leash walks.

3. Gizmo, a seven-year-old Shih Tzu, had a torn and ruptured Achilles tendon, causing him to have dropped hock. He was unable to have surgical repair of the rupture due to medical and financial reasons, so a custom tarsal wrap was used, with crisscrossed elastic straps placed behind the heel to help hold the hock up. This wrap provided a permanent functional solution for Gizmo's leash walks. If Gizmo had been a larger, heavier dog, a splint or brace might have been considered.

Reiki

West meets East! Physical therapy blends well with Eastern forms of medicine such as Reiki and acupuncture. Although PT is considered to be traditional medicine in the human field, it is complementary to many in the veterinary world. It can be combined beautifully with ancient forms of healing to produce optimum results without counterproductive effects.

If you have ever experienced Reiki, you probably found it relaxing and beneficial. I first became aware of Reiki from my human physical therapy patients, who had sought this type of treatment for medical issues. I was skeptical about it, until I entered the veterinary world and observed it being given to animals. I became intrigued and scheduled a session for myself.

The Reiki practitioner explained that the Reiki system of healing was lost for many centuries but rediscovered by Dr. Usui in the late 1800s. Dr. Usui was a religious teacher who had an enormous amount of scholarly and technical information about healing, but he lacked spiritual power or the ability needed to heal. He went on a twenty-one-day pilgrimage of meditation and fasting, where he lost consciousness and was filled with energy and healing powers. After this he began to heal many people in Japan and started to pass along his gift to other healers through ceremony and attunements. Reiki continues to be passed along to students who study and receive it and are attuned by a Reiki master.

My session consisted of lying on a table, fully clothed, while the practitioner placed her hands gently in various positions on and just above the body. The hands felt warm and sometimes even hot. She told me I might experience waves, vibrations, or see images and different colors. I asked her, "You mean like in the sixties?" (Just kidding, I had to say it!) Though I did not have any of those sensations, I did feel a deep relaxation and a sense of well-being.

This same practitioner worked with me at a shelter I service weekly and sensed that I had a natural healing energy. She said that being attuned to first level Reiki would be an added benefit or dimension to my skills as a physical therapist. There are three levels of Reiki, the first of which is a hands-on type;

the other two are at a distance level. I finally did receive attunement, after studying and receiving Reiki over the course of a few weeks. The attunement was a little freaky for me, being a Western, traditional type of medical professional, but I enjoyed the experience. It involved positions, hand placement, drinking water, contracting certain body areas, symbols drawn over me with the hand, etc. At the end there was a type of thumping on the top of my head, where the Reiki is supposed to enter you, but I honestly did not feel anything.

I had been advised to eat lightly and drink a lot of water the few days prior, as my body would want to cleanse itself afterward. I promptly ignored this advice, thinking it sounded a bit silly. Well, it wasn't so funny the next day when I was driving to a PT conference and I became in serious need of finding the nearest bathroom STAT. I will spare you the details, but just know I became a believer right then and there!

So, is Reiki for real? Well, my answer is: I don't know for sure, but I think so. I truly hope I am not offending any Reiki masters who might be reading this. I am just providing my own perspective as a novice. I do use first level Reiki during many PT sessions, usually after massage or trigger point releases. I lay my hands lightly on various places on the animal's body (using recommended placements and my intuition). I close my eyes and try to relax and just let the energy flow through me. My hands feel warm and sometimes tingly. The animals usually always love it! They get very relaxed and other pets in the house become quiet and still. Whether it is Reiki, the Holy Spirit, my love for animals, or all of the above, it seems to be very effective.

I've also seen some amazing effects of Reiki treatment given by the master practitioner I work with at the shelter. One time was in the medical recovery, when she stood outside of the cages where animals were coming out of anesthesia from spay/ neuter or other surgery. With her hands raised in the direction of the animals, I would observe the initial whining and crying from the semi-conscious animals start to wane and even stop when she started flowing Reiki toward them. They couldn't see her but they obviously sensed her presence or the Reiki energy or both, and it comforted them. Another time involved some injured cougars that arrived at the zoo from Texas, who were anxious and aggressive. The Reiki master gave them distance energy from the other side of the barn, through thick walls, and they became quieter and calmer.

So, it seems there is some evidence that Reiki is "real." I understand it from a biofield perspective, where charged particles in atoms produce currents of energy on and around the body surface. I don't have an understanding of chakras, etc., but respect those who have this knowledge. Health practitioners working with animals need to keep an open mind regarding Reiki and other holistic forms of healing, for the benefit of an animal's health and well-being.

Acupuncture

For over 4,000 years, Chinese acupuncture has been in use for a variety of medical conditions. In the eighteenth century, it expanded into the realm of animal health. In the mid-1970s, the International Acupuncture Society was formed and acupuncture began to be integrated into Western veterinary science and training. Currently in the United States, animal acupuncture is performed primarily by licensed veterinarians who receive additional certification. They are generally referred to as "integrative veterinarians." Some states may have laws that allow other practitioners to become licensed or certified in the practice of acupuncture on animals. As a general rule, physical therapists do not perform acupuncture, unless their particular state allows it.

Acupuncture is used to restore and balance the flow of chi, or vital life energy, which circulates through the body along linear pathways or energy channels called "meridians." Some Western practitioners refer to chi as "bioelectric force." Along the meridians are precise acupuncture points that are stimulated by needles that are inserted and manipulated for the purpose of freeing blocked chi flow. There are fourteen meridians in animals, twelve associated with body organ systems (lung, intestine, stomach, bladder, kidney, liver, gall bladder, etc.), and two on the body midlines (along the spine and belly, lengthwise). Individual acupuncture points are named by pairing a number with the meridian.

Acupuncture is used to maintain health, prevent illness, and treat medical conditions. It can help animals absorb nutrients, boost their immune system, improve respiration, reduce seizures, relieve pain, manage stress, etc. Acupuncture is immensely valuable and offers alternatives to traditional health management, especially in cases where medications are not effective or tolerated.

Acupuncture can be provided as an alternative to physical therapy or in conjunction with it. My professional opinion is that the acupuncturist is the best person to determine if physical therapy should be performed at the same time, or stopped until acupuncture treatment concludes. I base this on the fact that the two methods work on fundamentally different philosophies and may impact each other negatively. Some acupuncture treatments require a period of rest and refraining from vigorous activity, thus physical therapeutic exercise programs may interfere with or reduce the potential benefit of acupuncture.

In contrast to acupuncture is a treatment performed by specially trained physical therapists called "dry needling." Although it uses the same type of needle as acupuncture, a solid filament needle, it is an entirely different intervention and not based on ancient Chinese medicine. Dry needling is used with trigger points to relax muscles, based on theory and treatment developed by Dr. Janet Travell in the 1950s.

Stem Cell Procedures

The field of regenerative medicine is growing (no pun intended), at a rapid rate, especially in veterinary practice. Although there is no hard evidence as to the short- and long-term effects of this new science, its future is promising. Using cells and cell tissue, the goal of these procedures is to stimulate and enhance healing. Physical therapy, which shares a common goal of helping the body heal itself, is a logical adjunct to stem cell procedures.

Stem cell procedures are used to treat arthritic joints, meniscus cartilage tissue, and even ligaments or tendons. Adult (somatic) stem cells are used, instead of embryonic stem cells. These cells are taken from fat tissue, which is removed from the animal's body while under anesthesia. The harvested tissue gets processed, using a culture and expansion method to refine and isolate stem cells. This processing phase can take forty-eight hours to two weeks, depending on the method used. Some highly specialized institutions have the ability to perform this on-site, in an hour or so. Afterward, the stem cells are injected, directly into the affected joints or tissue or into the bloodstream, under sedation.

Once implanted, the stem cells work to enhance regeneration potential of damaged tissue and restore function. Physical therapy, by use of modalities such as laser and low intensity electrical current, provides mechanical stimulation to help the stem cells integrate into the tissue being treated. In a sense, PT plays a proactive role in targeting mechanical stimuli to help train the implanted cells how to behave.

These modalities, along with gentle range of motion exercises, are typically started twenty-four to forty-eight hours after the procedure. Range of motion exercises can be performed two to three times per day, along with slow leash walks of short, five-minute durations. The duration of leash walks is progressed to ten minutes during the next week or so and ultimately progressed according to the veterinarian's recommendations. No running, jumping, or playing should be allowed until weeks after the procedure. Laser and electrical stimulation modalities can be provided two to three times per week the first week, then one to two times per week.

At the present time, the stem cell implants are expensive and considered experimental by many insurance carriers. Continual advances and developments take place with this exciting field, including treatment of neural tissue in cases of paralysis and the extraction of cells from olfactory tissue to aide in other types of regeneration. The future of stem cell regenerative medicine will hopefully encompass organ disease as well.

(See Note 21.)

Chiropractic

I am often asked if physical therapists are against the work of chiropractors, or dislike them. My answer is "No way!" Many physical therapists respect and value the role of chiropractors in the medical field, both human and veterinary. In fact, there are many areas in which the two fields overlap: in performing spinal mobilizations and manipulations, applying modalities like electrical stimulation, and various types of stretching exercises. The main difference is in philosophy and fundamental principles of chiropractic, which is where physical therapists part ways. The chiropractic field embraces the theory that misaligned or subluxed vertebrae in the spinal column interrupt nerve signals and cause a variety of ailments. The obvious ones are pinched nerves that can cause tingling and pain, or stiffness and blocked movements in the back. Less obvious ailments that chiropractors believe are caused by subluxation include immune system, bladder, liver, and organ disturbances. Physical therapists, along with most mainstream medical professionals, believe that many systems in the body work relatively independent of the spinal nerves. For example, the circulatory system, and various hormones that are produced to help regulate body functions and organ systems, outside of the influence of the spinal column.

Many human patients, who use chiropractors regularly and proactively, claim to have improved immune systems and overall health because of these treatments. Perhaps it is from the alignment of vertebrae or simply a result of a pleasant experience that reduces stress and therefore helps boost natural immune function. I don't claim to know, but I do admire and respect the positive results I have seen in patients receiving chiropractic care.

Chiropractic care is generally very affordable and often has quick results, especially in acute stages of an injury, particularly in the spine. The down side is that the results may not be long-lasting and might require multiple repeat visits. Some chiropractors promote long-term dependence on having regular adjustments. Adjustments are made manually with the doctor's hands or using an instrument called an "activator."

Chiropractors who receive special training can utilize a patented technique called "Active Release" (ART), where the patient performs a prescribed movement while the chiropractor applies a pressure or tension to relieve overused muscles.

The best criteria to use in choosing a chiropractor to help your pet are that the doctor is a member of American Veterinary Chiropractic Association (AVCA) or has been trained in animal anatomy and treatment. The doctor should be working exclusively with animals, or have a separate office or space in which animals are treated, with distinct hours of operation apart from his or her human practice. This has more to do with mindset and concentrating focus on the unique anatomy and bodily structures on animals rather than public relations or health facility standards (though these are important too).

Overall, any chiropractor working with animals should consider his or her role as an adjunct to traditional veterinary care. As with physical therapy, chiropractic is not a substitution for the regular care your pet's veterinarian provides.

I Might Have No Business Saying This *But…*

I hope by this point in the book I have earned the right to speak my mind about a few things that may be of help. Well, here goes:

1.   Euthanasia: When it is your pet's "time" and the decision is made to euthanize, please, please summon all of your strength and courage to be present for the event. You will never regret it. If you don't stay with your pet, you will surely regret not being there afterward. Your presence, your hands on the pet's head or body, your voice, your

calmness, and your prayers or spiritual feelings will be of great help to your pet during the procedure. Just smile at it through your tears and tell your pet it's been a good companion and friend, and all will be well.

2. On the afterlife: Do I think animals go to heaven, or have a soul, or that we will see them in another life? *Yes.*

3. Don't create a sick pet: For some weird reason, there are folks who just seem to enjoy being sick, focusing on their symptoms or anything negative, making excessive visits to the doctor or therapist, usually for a secondary gain, I suppose. I saw it plenty in my human physical therapy days. Please don't do this to your pet. Animals do not want to be sick and if we focus too much on this, they may become passive, aggressive, or display mental or behavioral changes. Our pets tend to model us and are sensitive to our habits and feelings. We are a strong source of information for them and they read us intently. It is best to focus our time and energy on keeping a positive approach to their health care: being proactive, practicing preventative measures, and staying focused on moving quickly from sick mode to recovery mode when illness or injury occurs.

4. On visiting animal shelters: Unless you are actively looking for a pet to adopt, a visit to the animal shelter is not easy but important. Please don't use the excuse: "I can't go because I would want to bring all of them home with me." Nearly everyone uses this excuse and it is a real yawn and eye roller. It is good to visit your local shelter

and bring along a donation, see the animals, and show your support. It also keeps the staff and management on their toes, when the public shows interest and presence. The animals in the shelter do not want to be pitied; they want you to acknowledge them.

5. On groomers: Keep your pet groomed during its rehabilitation, especially for nail trimming and hair clipping. Find a groomer who will not confine your pet in a cage for lengthy periods if at all, and who provides a fun, low-stress environment for the animal. Let him or her know that your pet is undergoing physical therapy and has special needs in terms of handling and positioning. A good groomer who is an expert and passionate about his or her craft will take the necessary time and attention to make modifications to ensure your pet stays safe and comfortable.

6. On Tellington Touch, pet massage, and the like: they can be helpful and effective, but are not substitutes for the skills and education of a physical therapist. These services might be very beneficial after physical therapy is completed. I don't recommend having your pet undergo these services in tandem with physical therapy as it may be too much hands-on care and interfere with the desired effects of treatment. The exception to this is Reiki, which seems to enhance and blend well with physical therapy. Be sure to check the credentials and training of every practitioner and ensure that they work exclusively or predominately with animals, not just on the side as a hobby.

Final words: My true hope for this book is to help our pets by empowering their consumers through knowledge and guidance. When you approach your pet's health care from a position of strength and being informed, you have an advantage in making decisions and interacting with your pet's veterinarian, therapist, and other professionals. You are a savvy, wise, and concerned pet owner who will secure the best health outcome for your precious animal!

Appendix

Helpful Resources

Organizations
American Physical Therapy Association: www.apta.org
Orthopaedic Section/APTA's Animal Rehabilitation Special Interest Group:
www.orthopt.org/sig_apt.php
International Association of Veterinary Rehabilitation and Physical Therapy:
www.iavrpt.org
Veterinary European Physical Therapy and Rehabilitation Association:
http://www.vepra.eu/
Association of Chartered Physiotherapists in Animal Therapy: www.acpat.org
Veterinary Chiropractors: www.avcadoctors.com
National Board of Certification for Animal Acupressure and Massage:
www.nbcaam.org

Blogs
Dawg Business (by Jana Rade): http://dawgbusiness.blogspot.com
Fidose of Reality (by Carol Bryant): www.fidoseofreality.com
Dr. Patrick Mahaney, VMD: www.patrickmahaney.com

Educational Programs
University of Tennessee's Canine and Equine Rehabilitation Program:
www.canineEquineRehab.com
Canine Rehabilitation Institute: www.caninerehabinstitute.com
Tallgrass Animal Acupressure Institute: www.animalacupressure.com

Finding Health Care Providers
Land of PureGold Foundation's Canine Physical Therapy Assistance:
http://landofpuregold.com/challenge-physical.htm
TopDog's Canine Rehabilitation Directory: http://topdoghealth.com/
Canine-Rehabilitation-Directory/

Support and Products

Handicapped Pets: http://www.handicappedpets.com/index.php/leg-splints.html
Your Active Pet: http://www.youractivepet.com
Scout's House: http://www.scoutshouse.com
DoggLeggs: http://www.dogleggs.com/files/products.cfm
Walkabout Harnesses: http://www.walkaboutharnesses.com
Doggie Essentials: http://www.doggieessentials.com
Able Pet: http://ablepet.com
Toe Grips: http://www.toegrips.com
Eddie's Wheels: http://eddieswheels.com
The Help 'Em Up Harness: http://helpemup.com
Go Pet: www.gopetusa.com

Braces and Splints

My Pet's Brace: http://www.mypetsbrace.com/rear-leg-orthotic-braces.php
K-9 Orthotics and Prosthetics: http://www.k-9orthotics.com/orthotics/
    stifle-orthosis
Thera-Paw: http://www.therapaw.com
Ace Ortho Solutions: http://www.aceorthosolutions.com
Ortho Vet: http://orthovet.com

Books

Canine Physical Therapy: Orthopedic Physical Therapy, by Deborah M. Gross,
    MSPT, OCS, Wizard of Paws, 2002
Canine Rehabilitation and Physical Therapy, by Darryl L. Millis, David Levine,
    and Robert A. Taylor, Saunders, First Edition 2004, Second Edition 2013
Control of Canine Genetic Diseases, by George A. Padgett, DVM, Howell Book
    House, 1998

Notes

1. http://healthypets.mercola.com/sites/healthypets/archive/2010/02/03/benefits-of-physical-therapy-for-dogs.aspx

2. http://www.ibizan.freeservers.com/assessin.htm

3. http://www.josr-online.com/content/5/1/1

4. http://veterinarypage.vetmed.ufl.edu/2011/09/19/laser-treatment-helps-dogs-with-spinal-cord-injury/

5. http://www.bellevuemassagetherapy.com/scar-tissue-massage.html

6. http://corgicare.com /a-dog-workout-exercises-and-activities/

7. http://trace.tennessee.edu/cgi/viewcontent.cgi?article=1402&context=utk_chanhonoproj&sei-redir=1&referer=http%3A%2F%2Fwww.google.com%2Furl%3Fsa%3Dt%26rct%3Dj%26q%3Dresearch%-2520studies%2520on%2520underwater%2520treadmills%2520for%-2520animals%26source%3Dweb%26cd%3D4%26ved%3D0CD0QFjAD%26url%3Dhttp%253A%252F%252Ftrace.tennessee.edu%252Fcgi%252Fviewcontent.cgi%253Farticle%253D1402%-2526context%253Dutk_chanhonoproj%26ei%3DFY6uUaG7Erai4A-Ok5IDQBw%26usg%3DAFQjCNF6D5dHFG8Lt8kiCBBRwNcj_kBy-cQ%26bvm%3Dbv.47380653%2Cd.dmg#search=%22research%20studies%20underwater%20treadmills%20animals%22

8. http://www.google.com/#sclient=psy&hl=en&q=center+of+gravity+and+base+of+support+in+canines&aq=&aqi=&aql=&oq=center+of+-gravity+and+base+of+support+in+canines&pbx=1&fp=5fc6e4edb7c346e

9. http://www.ncbi.nlm.nih.gov/pubmed/17546211

10. http://www.whole-dog-journal.com/issues/13_2/features/canine-Ligament-Injury-Options_16198-1.html

11. http://dawgbusiness.blogspot.com/2010/02/acl-injuries-in-dogs-non-surgical.html

12. http://en.wikipedia.org/wiki/Comparative_foot_morphology

13. http://www.ivis.org/journals/vetfocus/21_2/en/1.pdf

14. http://pets.webmd.com/dogs/dog-wound-care-treatment?page=2

15. http://www.caninefitness.com/docs/Conservative-Rx-IVDD.pdf

16. https://smartech.gatech.edu/bitstream/handle/1853/14741/presentation_forest.pdf

17. http://veterinarynews.dvm360.com/dvm/Medicine/canine-rehabilitation-evolving-to-aid-arthritic-po/ArticleStandard/Article/detail/622213

18. http://www.akcchf.org/canine-health/your-dogs-health/canine-athlete/athlete-health-resouces.html

19. http://www.dogarthritisblog.info/dog-joint-health-1/walking-with-your-dog-a-fun-and-cheap-form-of-dog-physical-therapy

20. http://www.ncbi.nlm.nih.gov/pubmed/2975277

21. http://www.petmd.com/blogs/fullyvetted/2011/feb/stem_cell_therapy_debate

Index